Natural Health
for Women

Other books by Belinda Grant Viagas

The Detox Diet Book
A–Z of Natural Healthcare
Natural Remedies for Common Complaints

ACKNOWLEDGEMENTS

Nora Viagas, my mother and friend, was a source of endless inspiration and encouragement, and the thread of her wisdom weaves through every page.

Gordon Scott Wise, Senior Editor at Boxtree/ Macmillan, helped shape the book with his excellent suggestions and great sense of form.

Tina Betts and her team at Andrew Mann were always there with friendly support and advice whenever I needed them.

I value Mark Reidy and his sage comments, friendship and care.

My thanks to Judy Love and 'Ginger' for their presence towards the end, and of course to Amy.

Advice to the Reader

Before following any medical, dietary or exercise advice contained in this book, it is recommended that you consult your doctor if you suffer from any health problems or special conditions or are in any doubt as to its suitability.

Natural Healthcare for Women

BELINDA GRANT VIAGAS
ND, DO, DipC

newleaf

First published in Great Britain 1997 by Newleaf,
an imprint of Macmillan Publishers Ltd,
25 Eccleston Place, London, SW1 9NF and Basingstoke.

Associated companies throughout the world

ISBN 0 7522 05781

Jacket design by Slatter-Anderson
Illustrations by Cath Knox
Cover photograph: © Bokelberg/Image Bank

1 3 5 7 9 10 8 6 4 2

A CIP catalogue entry for this book is available from the
British Library

Typeset by SX Composing DTP, Rayleigh, Essex
Printed and bound in Great Britain by
Mackays of Chatham plc, Chatham, Kent

CONTENTS

INTRODUCTION

Natural healthcare is a complete system that is elegant in its simplicity. Its philosophy is that the body's own intelligence requires nurturing and support to achieve its own goal of perfect health. It recognises that every individual has both a different prescription for full health, and makes a different journey to get there. Natural healthcare truly treats the person, and not the symptoms or the disease. By strengthening the constitution, reinforcing the immune system and encouraging the body's own abilities to digest and eliminate, resistance to disease is increased along with energy levels, vitality and general well-being.

Happiness, our ability to relax, the success of relationships and our sense of ease with ourselves are all vital factors in our quest for health. We can directly influence our lives, and our health, by the way we spend our days, the amount of outdoor contact we have, and whether we honour those things that are sacred to us.

Natural healthcare embraces a wealth of remedies and measures to promote full health and well-being, from the simplest relaxation skills to the use of herbs and medicinal foods. Women have traditionally had an affinity with this gentle and immediate form of healing that includes plants, herbal remedies and physical care. In mediaeval days many of these guardians of nature's lore were burned as witches, and often their only crime was in being midwives or nature cure practitioners. As nurturers and carers our connection with the healing powers of foods, herbs, comfort and care was learned in a very real way, and this is what has brought our species this far.

Natural measures can enrich our lives throughout all their changing seasons. We live so close to the magic and mystery of our experience, and can journey smoothly through the transitions and challenges with gentle support and encouragement that will enhance our health naturally.

We cannot divorce our thoughts, dreams and desires from the way our body works, or from the spirit that animates and inspires us. The way we feel emotionally directly influences the way we feel physically, and vice versa. It makes good sense, therefore, to include psychological factors alongside physical measures in our own healthcare plans, and to embrace and make time for the sacred in our lives.

Cultivating a sense of peace within ourselves, the ability to relax and let go of stresses, and the capacity for happiness are all as vital as more medicinal measures. To effect our own well-being means honouring our need for self-expression as much as we need to ensure good nutrition. Enjoying full health means experiencing happiness and contentment. We can't be totally well if we are worried, over-stressed, bored or unhappy. Our mental outlook has every bit as much of an impact on our well-being as do the foods we eat and the genes we were born with.

This blend of measures makes for a form of healthcare, or a way of living, that fully embraces all aspects of our lives, and searches out quality in all that we do.

Developing the many different aspects of ourselves enriches and fulfils us in myriad ways. Creativity, intuition, sensuality, strength and all the other qualities that make us who we are need expression just as our muscles need exercise.

As women we have a finger on the pulse of the future, and a strong connection with each other and with the natural world. When we allow the influence of the changing seasons and cycles into our awareness we enhance our daily lives beyond measure.

Sometimes spending some time gazing out of the window in the morning can be a good way to start the day and reinforce our place in the greater scheme of things. Seeing that the world outside reflects our own inner landscape offers an immediate connection with something bigger and greater than our own lives. Bringing that world indoors through the use of plants, herbs, flowers and other natural remedies touches us in a very immediate way.

These gifts from nature are always available to us, and by using their gentle effects to balance and heal our bodies we take part in something very special; a treatment without side effects that doesn't cause any pollution or destruction, and that doesn't harm any level of our experience. Better yet, one that enhances our innate strength and vitality and brightens the future for ourselves and for our children.

To embrace natural healthcare is to relax in the knowledge that we don't have to experience pain in order to gain, and that the medicine need not taste bitter. It cultivates an understanding that sometimes it is the simplest things that will make a difference, like taking a walk to relieve a stuffy headache. When more is needed, the answer is usually there in a herb or a tissue salt or in returning to a good health habit.

It is little wonder that we should look to the majesty and beauty of the natural world for our healing. We know we will find the power there to renew and revitalise us, and to settle any disharmony.

Looking after ourselves is also tremendously empowering, and we can do this in a way that brings harmony to our lives and our surroundings. We can choose to support our health and live our lives in ways that cultivate balance and do not harm others. From deciding not to give mental house room to malicious thoughts, to petitioning for the provision of safer foods, or buying locally grown produce, or ensuring that we spend some time in nature every day to remind us of our roots, all of these affect our day-to-day experience as directly as more targeted health measures. When we opt for a method of treatment that will reinforce our own beliefs, and support our journey towards full health, or adopt good health habits to anchor us in our busy world, then we take a stride towards embodying our own potential, and begin to experience 'walking our talk'.

Prevention of ill health is all about keeping our lives in balance. When we weigh our health needs against all the time constraints of modern living, something has to give, but if we develop the quality of all aspects of our life, then we have a recipe for full health and happiness.

CHOOSING NATURAL
HEALTHCARE

If Natural Healthcare is a whole new world to you, start gently. Begin by asking questions and thinking about the everyday assumptions that we all make about our health. We assume that the food we can buy is good for us, and that the water that comes through our taps is safe to drink; we often think that companies care and that government legislation is in place to safeguard our interests.

Most of the food in our shops is chemically grown, and treated with a vast array of synthetic factors from pesticides to fungicides, growth enhancers and finishes. Then it is likely to have been processed in some way – waxed or bottled, canned or frozen, with the addition of fillers, preservatives, flavourings and colourings. Some foods are completely denatured, have their chemical structure changed or their genes altered, or are routinely irradiated, and labelling is less than clear.

These foods that we eat should be providing our body with the energy for clear thought, ease of movement, and ongoing good health. It makes good sense to eat only the best possible foods, grown naturally and well, and offered to us in a way that we know is concerned with our nutrition and health, rather than with manufacturing profit levels and extended shelf life in mind.

We face a thousand choices every time we go out shopping, with the enormous variety of foods that are available to us. Everything is, in essence, a potential health giver, and we must ensure that this continues to be so by making the healthiest possible choices for ourselves and our families.

Beyond the riches of the greengrocers, it is well worth getting to know your local healthfood shop. Although many of the products that started life in these places are now to be found on supermarket shelves, there is still plenty of exploration to be done. Tofu, ghee and soya products can now all be found at supermarkets and grocery stores, but healthfood shops may offer you a wider choice of ranges and varieties, as well as being able to tempt you with other things that you may like to try.

Make changes slowly to your diet, your shopping experiences and your style of food preparation. One good way to achieve a healthier balance is to target any changes that you need to make, and focus on achieving one each week, or each month. Let yourself experiment with new foods to add richness to your diet and see if you develop any new favourites. In our society, wheat is used as a staple, and is found in an enormous number of foods. Explore other options including rice, potatoes, millet, corn, rye and mixed grains; it makes good health sense and is good for our taste buds too. Cows' dairy produce is another food that we rely on, and the full range of other milks, goats' and sheeps' yoghurts, and cheeses is well worth exploring. Grains are often used as the basis for alternative milks, and you will find ranges that are rice-, soya- and barley-based.

You do not need to peel most fruit and vegetables, unless they have been chemically grown. Many of the nutrients in vegetables, like the roughage and vitamins, lie in or just below the skin, and often a good scrub is all that is needed. If you do need to peel, pare very thinly.

Steam rather than boil foods, and grill rather than fry, this preserves flavour, nutrient levels, and cuts down on unnecessary fat. The amount and type of fat you eat is very important. Saturated fats come from animals in the main, and too much is unhealthy. It is heavy with energy in a form that is very difficult for the body to access and utilise, and it contributes to heart failure through its effect on the blood vessels. Fats that come from vegetable sources are still very rich in energy, but have a positive effect within the body. Look for cold-pressed oils that are simple extractions from the fruit or nut.

Wherever possible avoid vegetable margarines made from hydrogenated oils with an ingredient list that is as long as the packet – you are much better off eating small amounts of butter, or a spread containing no trans-fats or hydrogenated oils such as Vitaquell. Hydrogenated oils use up all your antioxidant vitamins (A, C and E) and contribute to the ageing process of every cell. They are only in existence to make manufacturing easier, and are entirely devoid of any nutritional value. Avoid them wherever possible.

Fats are clearly labelled in foods. Animal fat of marine origin means whale blubber. These magnificent creatures are far better left swimming through our oceans, and their addition to biscuits and pastries does nothing to enhance their flavour. It is also very hard for the body to digest.

Organically grown produce is well worth tasting. Often it will remind you of flavours from the past. I felt like an old lady the first time I found myself saying that 'I hadn't tasted an apple like that for years', but it was true! It is a lot better than chemically grown fruit and vegetables, although the cost and lack of availability can sometimes be prohibitive. Consider mixing your produce and having organically grown fruit and salad vegetables, and use others for cooking, or simply follow your budget and let seasonal availability dictate.

Start using sea salt for its greater iodine and mineral content, and use it sparingly – keeping it in the kitchen, not on the table, and using it only in cooking. Season your foods with herbs and spices, nature's own flavour enhancers.

Avoid additives, preservatives, monosodium glutamate (MSG), etc., and learn what E numbers are. As consumers we have a tremendous power to change the quality of foods for the better. Read the labels on everything, and reject anything that you don't trust. Your health is precious and you do not need to compromise.

Trawl the shelves of your healthfood shop and you will discover a range of seaweeds and sea vegetables. These are often used in Chinese and Japanese menus, so you can look there for inspired ideas for ways to use them, and recipes are always included on the labels. These are a valuable source of iodine and minerals that will boost metabolism, support thyroid function and help a host of other functions within the body. They also taste terrific, and are a wonderful way to add flavour and texture to soups and salads. Wakame is very good if rehydrated and snipped into salads. Nori is deliciously tasty and can be bought in dried sheets that you can use to wrap rice and other vegetables in, or it can be toasted and crumbled onto savoury dishes. Carageen can be ground and added to any meal, or used for its gelatinous qualities in sweets, fruit jellies and in place of aspic.

Tahini, halva and Gomasio are among a range of sesame seed products that are very tasty and a rich source of calcium. This is essential to women's health, particularly as we approach the menopause.

Tahini is creamed sesame seeds, and can be substituted for peanut butter, spread on toast, used to thicken sauces, or just dipped into. Halva is a sweet block form of sesame seeds that is often sweetened with honey and has pistachios, almonds or other nuts added. Gomasio is a flavouring made from sesame seeds and sea salt. It can be added to meals during cooking or at the table, and also makes a tasty coating for tofu or chicken.

Amongst the others seeds and nuts you will find sunflower and pumpkin seeds. These are very high in zinc and other necessary minerals, and make a tasty snack or topping for savoury dishes. Along with the tiny alfalfa seeds, these can all be sprouted to transform them into a living, nutritious food that is tasty and packed with vitamin C and protein. Place a selection of seeds or dried pulses (chick peas, mung beans, etc.) in a glass jar and rinse with warm water. Cover with a clean tea towel or some kitchen paper and leave on a windowsill in the kitchen. Repeat the warm water rinse two or three times each day, and within five days you will have a jar full of sprouts. You can buy a sprouter from most kitchen stores that will enable you to grow two or three tiers of sprouts at the same time just by watering two or three times a day.

Within the range of honeys you will find some that are enriched with pollen, propolis and Royal Jelly. These are all rich and valuable nutrients that have the effect of boosting overall health through their actions on the immune system. They are rich in antioxidants and have strong antifungal qualities too.

You will also find lots of dried fruit, and pulses. These differ from those you will find on the supermarket shelves in a few ways: they are likely to be unrefined, so you will see brown, wholewheat pasta rather than white, and pot barley, rather than the refined pearl. The fruits are likely to be stored in vegetable rather than mineral oil, and many will be without preservatives, so you will be able to find apricots that look the way you would expect them to rather than bright orange in colour.

Among the large range of products designed to offer an

alternative to wheat-based snacks, you will discover rice cakes. These look like polystyrene, yet their flavour makes them the perfect base for subtly flavoured toppings. Oatcakes and rye and soya flour form the base for other snack biscuits. Chewing these well releases the flavour, and is good advice generally.

Ancient texts speak of chewing each mouthful of food a requisite number of times to begin the work of digestion and fully satisfy the taste buds. Modern wisdom tells us that some processes actually begin in the mouth, like the breaking down of carbohydrates, so chewing is fundamentally important. It also contributes to the sensuous and gastronomic qualities of the meal.

Balance paying attention to your basic diet with regular treats and feasts. Food is a central part of any cure, but, once some sound habits have been established, it is necessary to free ourselves of any obsession or over-anxiety. One of the joys of a healthy diet such as this is that it will reduce stress levels, satisfy the taste buds, and mean that the body will begin to function healthily, so a range of minor health and weight complaints will disappear.

Achieving balance in our everyday lives means ensuring time for play as well as work, and leisure activities, exercise, socialising and private time are all necessary to maintain full health. Choosing natural healthcare means choosing to simplify your life from needless worries and interventions to a smooth-running source of energy and inspiration.

Working out your own individual recipe for full health means balancing your needs and desires with your expectations and existing obligations. The opportunity is always there for a complete overhaul of your health and your living habits, and nature is always there to support you in your own best efforts for health.

Getting the Best from This Book

This book is structured like a walk through a woman's life, beginning in childhood and then following the hormonal trail through to older age. Each chapter or event is a distinct time in a woman's life, although, as always, many of these will merge to become the rich tapestry that we experience as our daily reality.

Within each chapter you will find a discussion of the surrounding atmosphere along with ideas and suggestions to smooth any inconsistency or imbalance that could lead to ill health. Within each chapter, the section on Managing Change seeks to offer a range of options to strengthen the experience and transform any potentially negative or unhelpful aspects into positive, life-affirming aids. Your Body Now and What to Eat Now both deal with the physical changes that accompany each stage in life, and how best to meet them through nutrition and supplements. Exercises and activities, stretching routines and postures accompany dietary advice and food cures. A section on Staying Well completes each chapter with advice on natural remedies and healthcare measures to meet any associated health complaints. Case studies of women are included to illustrate the benefits of natural healthcare. Each chapter concludes with a small resource list of relevant further reading and useful addresses.

But first, the next chapter outlines some of the tools of natural healthcare and ways in which they can be used at home. This is followed by a chapter outlining how to choose a natural healthcare practitioner.

Finally, Your Natural Healthcare Plan includes tips on how to implement natural healthcare throughout your life.

TOOLS OF HEALING

Natural healthcare embraces a wealth of different therapies, practices, skills and techniques to support each individual fully in their move towards full health. What these all have in common is that none of them intervenes in the body's own processes, or interferes in any deleterious way. They seek to support and enhance or enable the body's own intelligence, and its best efforts to achieve optimum energy, vitality and balance.

Throughout this book you will find different ways of strengthening body systems, together with exercises to harness your energy and focus it on a specific outcome. These work alongside more familiar remedies and cures to ensure that every aspect of your full life is addressed. Some of the types of things you will find in this book are outlined here.

Attitude

By far the most important healing tool is our approach to health, our willingness to work and take pleasure in strengthening and refining the body, and our desire for healing. If we have an image of ourselves as strong, vital, happy, healthy women then we have the strongest ally. When we can visualise and imagine perfect health, then we have a template, a model from which to proceed. If we can see ourselves well in our mind's eye, and have the desire in our heart to make it so, then we have a powerful healing force within us.

9

All the tools that we can summon to help us in this task are easy to use and completely accessible. Whether we rely on meditation to centre ourselves, or a faith, or periods of reflection, all will have the desired effect if we invest our time and energy. The same is true for the use of affirmations, that brilliant tool that works so well at changing our preconceived ideas and habits, and all forms of visualisation.

When you close your eyes and daydream about being on holiday, or feeling good, you are using a very powerful tool that can also be used to support your health. Visualising the way you want your life to be gives you an internal model to work from. You can use this to strengthen your immune system, or to discover the best environment in which to live.

Affirmations seek to replace some of the negative or restrictive thoughts that may be wandering around your head, with more positive, effective, life-enhancing ones. Many of our ideas about our lives, and our health, are self-limiting, and we can use affirmations as a way to broaden our scope, and our sense of what we can achieve. Use these in a very general way, e.g. 'Today I am stronger than before', or 'I love my life', or to work with very specific complaints or issues. Repeat your affirmation as often as you remember it, writing it down each time you have a spare moment, so that you can read it as well as say it, and change it as often as you need. Make some time each day to combine visualising and actively affirming the type of future you want for yourself, and be sure to include specific health concerns.

When we are open to our lives being healed, and to the idea that we can play an active role in that process, then we begin truly to live our own lives. Imagine a life without happiness and joy, or without the comfort of good friends. When we reach out to improve the quality of our lives we enhance our health, every bit as much as by taking a remedy or eating a good meal. Health touches every aspect of our lives, and we can support and encourage that in a myriad ways.

Suggested reading
As I See It Betty Balcombe, Piatkus
Earth Medicine Kenneth Meadows, Element
Seven Arrows Hyemehosts Storm, Ballantine
All in the Mind Stephen Roet, Optima

Exercise

Exercise is one of the best all-round things we can do for our body, reminding it of natural rhythms, strengthening and stretching it, and producing natural mood enhancers.

Walking is one of the best all-round exercises, but it can only be done safely if care is taken to provide support. Appropriate footwear, a sports bra and cotton knickers and socks should ensure against most potential hazards. Walking is a weight-bearing exercise and as such is more important than other aerobic activities like swimming or cycling because it has been shown to have a protective effect against osteoporosis. It truly comes into its own as we approach our mid-thirties in preparation for the changes that accompany the menopause. It may seem like an early start, but this is the age when menstrual difficulties and other nutritional and hormonal changes begin to manifest themselves. In combination with either some form of press-up (proper ones, or done while sitting or standing and leaning forward) or weight training, it forms a complete workout for those years.

If you swing your arms while you walk you can increase the aerobic effect. Walking on hilly terrain will maximise its effect on your figure (shaping the waist, bottom and legs) and also its effect on your internal organs. It can amount to an internal massage as all your organs are routinely stretched and squeezed. This effect is also taking place on the gut, so bowel movements are encouraged, and this is one of the best cures I know for constipation.

Exercise needs to fit a number of criteria in order to be really useful. It should strengthen, encourage flexibility, have an aerobic capacity, and so an effect on the heart and lungs, and therefore the overall health, and be enjoyable.

Always seek to protect your body, and ensure that any equipment that you use is completely safe. If you run, or jog, always do so on a supportive surface that has some give in it like grass or tarmac. Do not run on concrete paving slabs – this injures just about every joint in the body. If part of your route needs to be over paving, use this to vary your speed and walk rather than run for that section. Ensure, too, that you use some form of shock-absorbing insole in your running shoes. Similarly, if you dance or do aerobic or step classes, make sure that the floor is properly sprung.

Sometimes specific exercises can be more useful than overall toning and a full body workout. If an area of your body has become restricted or strained, then remedial or educative exercises aimed at releasing and restoring full ease of function to that area will be most relevant.

Never push yourself beyond what feels comfortable when performing a particular exercise. If you can do it easily, increase the number of times you do it, rather than increasing the range or extent of any stretch or extension.

There are other forms of exercise that work with the body's more subtle energies. These all seek to enhance the Chi or vital energy within and around the body, and will be concerned with proper breathing as well as either holding postures (line in yoga) or making gentle, slow movements (like in T'ai Chi). Some Chi Kung warm-up exercises can be found on p.225-26, and these work to stretch and strengthen the energy pathways within the body. The Chi Dynamics exercises on p.228 combine gentle breathing with careful movement to enhance energy levels.

Suggested reading
Hard Bodies Gladys Portugues and Joyce Vedral, Thorsons
Vital Energy Jackie Young, Hodder & Stoughton

Essential Oils

Essential oils are extracted from herbs, woods and flowers and are an extremely potent way of using the concentrated active ingredients. Everything you experience through your sense of smell is processed by the body, in much the same way as the foods you eat. The aroma of the oils affects us directly through our sense of smell, and secondary effects will occur through any absorption through the skin. Aromatherapists use essential oils to massage the body.

The oils can be used exclusively for their scent and burned in special oil burners, or added to steam, or mixed into carrier oils and massaged into the body. At home they can also be mixed with a dispersant or carrier oil and added to the bath. Add two drops of essential oil of Jasmine or Rose for a luxurious hedonistic soak, or choose Bergamot or Geranium for something more uplifting. On occasions when you cannot bathe, add one drop of any oil to a hand or foot bath, and let that part soak in the perfumed water. Alternatively, add two drops to a little sesame or olive oil and use to massage yourself.

Thyme oil is a strong disinfectant with a real affinity for

the throat area, so burn this during the cold season when coughs and sneezes abound, or add a few drops to a radiator humidifier. Alternatively, add a few drops to a bowl of warm water, and wring a towel or tea-cloth out in it, then place on the radiator to infuse the whole room.

It is important to ensure the quality of the oils you use by buying from a reputable supplier. The oils are very potent and care needs to be taken that they are diluted as directed, and almost never applied neat to the skin. One exception is Ti-tree oil which can be applied directly to treat warts, verrucae and insect bites. Use a cotton bud to make sure that the surrounding area is not burned.

Essential oils that have particular affinity with women's conditions include:

- Rose, a powerful uterine tonic with an essentially feminine quality;
- Ylang-ylang, a strong aphrodisiac;
- Sandalwood, which will support kidney functions and is excellent for mature skins;
- Geranium, a naturally uplifting oil which will help regulate hormone levels;
- Clary Sage, to encourage period flow and regularity;
- Jasmine, the marvellous anti-depressant with strong sensuous overtones;
- Howood, a pelvic decongestant.

NB Certain essential oils need to be avoided in early pregnancy: Basil, Cinnamon, Clary Sage, Clove, Cypress, Fennel, Hyssop, Juniper, Marjoram, Myrrh, Oregano, Rose Maroc (Bulgar) and Thyme.

Good suppliers of essential oils include
Fragrant Earth PO Box 182, Taunton, Somerset TA1 1SD.
01823 335734

Aromatherapy Associates 68 Maltings Place, Bagleys Lane,
London SW6 2BY. 0171 731 8129

Verde Essential Oils 75 Northcote Road, Battersea, London
SW11. 0171 924 4379

Suggested reading
Aromatherapy: An A–Z Patricia Davies, C. W. Daniel

Food

Food is one of the most immediate ways that we can directly
influence our health. It is something that we work with
every day, and getting to know the medicinal and nutritive
values of foods can help us treat ill health, and promote
wellness.

We are all familiar with the basic food groups of proteins, fats and carbohydrates. Proteins build body tissue, and
are essential for all growth and repair. There are two main
distinctions, complete proteins which are mainly animal
based, and incomplete proteins. Complete proteins include
meat, fish, eggs, milk, yoghurt, cheese and soya. Incomplete
proteins include nuts, seeds, beans, pulses and grains, and
these need to be combined in order to make a complete
protein.

Fats enable many vitamins to be absorbed, provide
energy, insulation and protection and combine with protein
to form the cell walls. The different types are saturated,
mono-unsaturated, and poly-unsaturated. Saturated fats are

found in all animal produce, and also in refined oils, coconut and palm oils.

We need some saturated fat, but very little, in order to remain healthy. Mono-unsaturated fats have all the benefits of saturates, with few of the constraints, and can be found in nuts, seeds and olive oil. Poly-unsaturates are found in nuts and nut oils, fish and fish oils, and vegetable oils. They contain Essential Fatty Acids and can be taken in larger amounts. The proportion of fats in the overall diet should still be very low.

Carbohydrates are starch, sugar and fibre − essential for energy and healthy bowel function. Sources include whole grains, rice, pasta, potatoes, nuts, seeds, pulses and beans. Natural sugar sources are fruits and milk, and fibre is found in all vegetables, seeds, pulses and beans. These foods should make up the bulk of our diet.

Foods can also be classified according to the type of energy they provide. Root vegetables, for example, store their energy below the ground and can be very warming to the body. Vegetables grown above the ground are lighter in quality and impart that energy when eaten. The way we prepare foods also influences this − think about the warmth of a jacket potato, or a slow-cooked casserole, and the lighter energy of a stir-fry meal. We can use these qualities to treat ourselves on the simplest level: by eating soups and root vegetables when we have a cold, and need to warm the body; and by choosing light salad meals and juices to treat lethargy and heat exhaustion in the summer.

Foods can also be classified according to the effect they have in the body, e.g. black pepper, chilli and ginger are all hot, they heat the body and are useful for dispelling cold, stagnant complaints. They are best used in moderation because their effect is very strong. Cucumber, tofu, coriander seed and fennel are all cooling and will help dispel any heat from the body. These are useful in all festering conditions and in case of infection.

Eat warming spices like chilli, cloves or cayenne to make digesting meals easier. Add a little ginger powder to peanut butter or tahini to lighten the effect.

Foods can have especially sedating qualities like the effects of a warm milky drink before bedtime, or give an instant energy lift like a handful of raisins, or be cooling and refreshing like melon on a hot day.

Some foods contain large quantities of specific nutrients such as vitamins and minerals, and can be used as a medicine when needed. Other foods contain a host of medicinal qualities, like garlic which is antibiotic, antiviral and antibacterial, as well as having beneficial effects on the intestine, blood and the heart.

The taste of each food can do a lot to influence the body. When you bite a slice of lemon, the sour, acid taste has a puckering, astringent effect throughout the body, and the bitter taste of endive and tonic water will quieten the appetite. Sweet is a taste we all know, and, along with salty, is the most common.

Sweet is present throughout nature, we don't actually need to add sugar to foods – try for yourself to discern the sweet taste present in rice, milk, and some vegetables. It is the most satisfying of tastes, and the more refined our palates become, the more pleasure we are able to receive. Pungent completes the five major tastes, and good examples of this are basil, rosemary and watercress. It is a very complex taste, with a peppery-quality.

Every main flavour comprises elements of the others, and all tastes have an after-taste which also influences their effect on the body.

Not eating, and eating selectively, can also have a powerful effect upon us. The use of fasts and mono-diets is a wonderfully immediate way to give our digestive systems a rest and free up body energy for other tasks – like healing, or meeting an acute health crisis. Fasting can become a regular part of your health regime, and resting in this way for one day each week or month will have a rejuvenating and energy-boosting effect on your whole system. The simplest way to do this is to drink only large amounts of water for a full twenty-four hours, and then return to a normal diet the next day. It is rather like having a day off, and is quite a safe and natural thing for the body to do – this is often what you are being urged to do in response to illness, for instance when you lose your appetite with the first sign of a cold or 'flu.

A gentler way to start, if fasting is new to you, is to spend a day on a fruit fast, or a juice fast. Choose a fruit that you like, and eat only that all day – pears, apples and grapes are a good and easy choice, or you may decide on pineapple for its excellent detox benefits, or mangoes just because. Make sure to drink lots of water as well as eating the fruit, and enjoy.

Suggested reading

Natural Remedies for Common Complaints Belinda Grant Viagas, Piatkus

The Ayurvedic Cookbook Arabella Morningstar, Lotus Press

A–Z of Health Foods Carol Bowen, Hamlyn

E for Additives M. Hanssen, Thorsons

Superfoods Michael van Straten and Barbara Griggs, Dorling Kindersley

The Ethical Consumer Guide ECRA Publishing (Manchester)

Back to Balance Dylana Accolla with Peter Yates, Newleaf

Perfect Health Deepak Chopra, Bantam

Further information
Incorporated Society of British Naturopaths Kingston, The Coach House, 293 Gilmerton Road, Edinburgh EH16 5UQ. 0131 664 3435

British Society for Nutritional Medicine PO Box 3AP, London 3AP 1MN. 0171 436 8532

Movement for Compassionate Living 47 Highlands Road, Leatherhead, Surrey KT22 8NQ

Flower Remedies

Flower Remedies are the essences of a variety of flowers that have been steeped in water, potentised or activated by sunlight, and often then preserved in alcohol. They seem to have a particular affinity with the more subtle energies of the body and are an effective way to address emotional and energetic imbalance. They can either be taken as a few drops on the tongue or drunk in a small glass of water or by direct application to the skin around the pulse spots (i.e. on the wrists, behind the knees, and behind the ears). Take first thing in the morning, last thing at night, and at least once or twice during the day, more if possible.

When a mix of remedies is desired, add the required number of drops to a small bottle of still mineral water and keep it in the fridge. This can then be drunk or applied easily at intervals through the day.

Rescue Remedy is a mix of remedies that is an excellent first-aid measure. Take or apply to soothe shock, nerves, and physical and emotional pain. When used for physical trauma it can shift the focus towards other means of expression, so your fingers will stop hurting, but you might start to cry. Like all flower remedies it can be added to a compress and placed over an area to soothe and treat.

Dr Bach Flower Remedies is the range most often recommended in this book because it is the range most widely available in the UK. This is now being manufactured mechanically. Other ranges are still naturally based and produced, and include Australian Bush Remedies and Californian Gem Remedies. These can be bought at health-food shops and good pharmacies.

Recommended reading
A Guide to Bach Flower Remedies Julian Barard, C. W. Daniel
The Encyclopedia of Flower Remedies Clare Harvey with Amanda Cohrane, Thorsons

Further information
Dr Bach's Flower Remedies The Edward Bach Centre, Mount Vernon, Sotwell, Wallingford, Oxon OX10 OPZ. 01491 839489
International Flower Essence Repertoire The Working Tree, Milland, Nr. Liphook, Hampshire GU30 7JS. 01428 741572
Flower Essence Society PO Box 459, Nevada City, California 95959, USA. 001 800 548 0075

Herbs

Herbs have always been a mainstaff of healing. Adding them to the diet and taking them as teas are two simple and effective ways to experience their immediate benefits. Most fresh herbs can be chopped and added to salads, sandwiches and cooked meals. Experiment with adding some finely chopped horseradish flowers to sandwiches for a tasty treat that is rich in vitamins. Sprinkle some fresh cowslip flowers on salads to add potassium, vitamin A and a range of other minerals. Add thyme, rosemary and sage to cooking for their delicious flavours and their antibacterial qualities.

Drying is a convenient way of storing herbs, and can concentrate their flavour. In the main it does not damage the therapeutic value, and dried herbs can often be used interchangeably with fresh. They can be made into a tea by steeping in hot water. Chamomile is a popular after-dinner choice because of its digestion-enhancing qualities. Fennel and peppermint are also good choices with similar qualities. Lemon balm is a wonderfully refreshing and soothing tea that is delightful if made fresh on a summer's day. Add a few fresh borage flowers or some finely chopped borage leaf for a lovely cucumber-type flavour that will also be good for nutrient and relaxant levels.

Most of the common culinary herbs can be used in this way, and the less well-known herbs tend to be used more for their medicinal benefits, e.g. yarrow to support the kidneys and help with cystitis, and Lady's mantle to benefit the reproductive organs and ease menopausal symptoms. Most herbs are rich in vitamins and minerals, and are sometimes recommended for that sole purpose, e.g. parsley for its high levels of vitamin C and iron.

Herbs can also be used externally and their active ingredients absorbed through the skin. Made into creams and oils they can be applied whenever there is a need for immediate relief. As poultices and compresses their healing properties are instantly accessible.

- Make a strong walnut leaf tea or infusion, and use as a wash to cleanse an area of skin.

- Cut a fresh aloe leaf and apply directly to soothe irritated or burned skin.
- Rub a fresh dock leaf on the skin to relieve nettle stings.
- Use fresh lavender or tansy as a short-term insect repellent.
- Rub sweet-smelling herbs like rosemary and thyme to perfume your hands.

Wrap some herbs in a cotton handkerchief and tie to the tap when running a bath to allow their essence to infuse the bathwater. Oats are good for soothing troubled skin, lavender flowers will impart a wonderful sense of relaxation, and sage leaves will help lift you when tired and fatigued.

Tinctures are the herb's active ingredients distilled in alcohol. These can be taken directly under the tongue, or in a small glass of water. If the alcohol is not desired, rub onto the pulse spots on the wrists, neck and behind the knees (see page 19). Tinctures can be bought from some healthfood shops, herbal suppliers, and most herbalists.

Among the herbs you will find often used in this book are: sage, rosemary, mint, borage, thyme, chamomile, calendula and Lady's mantle.

NB Certain herbs should not be taken in therapeutic doses in early pregnancy: rue, golden seal, juniper, crocus, mistletoe, beerberry, pennyroyal, poke root, southernwood, wormwood, mugwort, tansy, nutmeg, cotton root, thuja, calendula, beth root, feverfew and sage.

Good herbal suppliers include

Potters Herbal Supplies, Leyland Mill Lane, Wigan WN1 2SB. 01942 34761

G. Baldwin and Co. 171 Walworth Road, London SE17 1RW. 0171 703 5550

Recommended reading
Kitty Campion's Handbook of Herbal Health Kitty Campion,
Sphere

Contact
The Herb Society 134 Buckingham Palace Road, London
SW1W 9SA. 0171 823 5583

Supplements

Many vitamins and minerals that are necessary for optimum
health are no longer to be found in our diet. This is because
so little of our food is grown naturally any more, most of what
we eat being chemically produced. This alters the nutrients
that the foods can make available to us. Also, many vitamins
and minerals are lost in storage and transportation – a few
hours out of the ground is half a lifetime for a delicate plant.
If we then cook them and further compromise their delicate
cell walls, or boil them and throw away the water, the
amount of active ingredient we are left with can be minimal.
The demands, stresses, and pollutants of modern life also
make greater tolls on the body's resources than ever before,
so we have a need for optimum nutrition.

Supplements can be broad based, or specific, and the
ingredients and sources must always be identified on the label.
Take care to avoid synthetic colourings, flavourings, preservatives and additives in these, as in everything that you take.
A good multivitamin and mineral supplement is good insurance at times of stress and change. For many of us, living busy
lives, this can mean much of the time. I always recommend
spending some time away from general supplementation, and
this is best done during the summer months. Individual vita-

mins or minerals may be taken as and when needed, e.g. extra vitamin C when you feel a cold coming on. Most often these can be taken with a meal, although some need to be taken away from food, and this is always mentioned on the label.

Supplements may be suggested in much higher doses by your practitioner, but for home use there are recommended minimum levels of many vitamins and minerals, and this is the information to look for on the product label. It is known in its abbreviated form as RDA and you will often see amounts represented as a percentage of the RDA or recommended daily allowance. Obviously, individual health needs vary, and will change from time to time, including throughout the menstrual cycle (blood loss with each period depletes iron reserves) and in response to seasonal factors (we need more nutrients when it's cold). Several vitamins and minerals have been shown to be essential during pregnancy to ensure adequate nutrition for both mother and foetus, e.g. folic acid. Lifestyle also plays a big factor, e.g. stress burns up B-vitamins, and both drinking coffee and smoking deplete chromium levels within the body. All nutritional factors influence each other, so care needs to be taken not to take too much of any one substance in isolation, or for too long a time without professional guidance.

Vitamins and minerals are quantified using different values, so some may be represented as micrograms (mcg), some as milligrams (mg), and some as International Units (IU).

The standard minimum daily requirements for common vitamins and minerals are:

Vitamins: vitamin A 2,500IU; vitamin B-complex – varies as per vitamin: vitamin B1 (thiamine) 10mg; B2 (riboflavin) 5mg; B3 (niacin/nicotinic acid) 10mg; B5 (pantothenic acid) not yet agreed; B6 (pyridoxine) 2mg; B12 (cyanocobalamin) 50mcg; biotin 150–300mcg; choline a maximum of 650mg;

inositol not yet agreed but likely to be around 1,000mg; folic acid 0.4mg; PABA (para amino benzoic acid) not yet agreed, likely to be around 100mg; vitamin C 30mg; vitamin D (cholecalciferol) 100IU; vitamin E (tocopherol) 30IU.

Minerals: calcium, 500mg; copper, less than 1 mg; iodine, 200mcg; iron is completely variable, e.g. a woman commonly loses 15–30mg with each period; magnesium, 150-450mg; manganese, 2mg; phosphorus 1.5–2mg; potassium, 2–4mg; selenium, 150mcg; sodium, 2mg; zinc, 15mg.

You tend to get what you pay for with vitamin and mineral supplements, although this is not exclusively so. One very well-publicised brand of expensive supplements is high in sugar substitutes, and low in essential vitamins. It is well worth consulting your practitioner, or taking the list above with you when shopping. Remember too, that you do not need sugar or its substitutes, colourings, flavourings, or any other synthetic additives in a supplement that is intended to do you good. You may also choose to seek out non-gelatine capsules and natural tableting ingredients.

All vitamins and minerals have quite complex actions within the body, and they interact with each other in a number of ways, e.g. zinc is essential for the release of vitamin A from the liver, vitamin D increases absorption of calcium from the diet, and vitamin B12 is essential to iron metabolism.

A brief guide to their activities and good food sources shows the benefits of eating a diet that is rich with variety:

* *Vitamin A* is concerned with the skin and eyes, and the maintenance of healthy mucous membranes. It can be found in all the yellow flowers, fruits and vegetables, including apricots, carrots, corn, squashes, pumpkins, and is also present in large amounts in violet leaves, dandelion

buds, papaya, watercress, spearmint, lettuce, chicory, oily
fish and dairy foods.

- *Vitamin B-complex* is a family of vitamins that all work
  together extremely closely within the body, and are found
  in similar sources in nature: yeast, green vegetables,
  especially broccoli, nuts and seeds, whole grains, eggs, and
  some seafood. These are the stress-buster vitamins that
  help strengthen the nerves and improve sleep.
- *Vitamin C* is responsible for the health of every cell and
  blood vessel in the body, and adds to healthy bone
  growth, wound healing and maintenance of gums and
  teeth. It is delicate and is destroyed by air, heat, light,
  metals and alkaline substances, which is why such great
  care needs to be taken to ensure a regular supply, and why
  raw foods are important in the diet. It is found in parsley,
  blackcurrants, broccoli and other green vegetables, citrus
  fruit, and potatoes. Take to speed healing, or to strengthen
  and reinforce the immune system in response to the threat
  of colds and 'flu.
- *Vitamin D* is essential to the formation of teeth and bones,
  and works with calcium and phosphorus to ensure their
  health. It can be made by the body through the activity of
  sunlight on the skin. In foods it can be found in small
  amounts in eggs, dairy produce, sunflower seeds and oily
  fish. Spend some time out of doors every day to maintain
  minimum levels within the body.
- *Vitamin E* is essential to fertility and muscle health, and
  along with vitamins A and C it is an anti-ageing agent.
  Find it in extra virgin olive oils, and also sunflower,
  grapeseed, wheatgerm, coconut and rapeseed oils. Take to
  facilitate ease of movement, and when feeling a bit creaky.
- *Vitamin K* is produced by the body and essentially keeps us
  from bleeding to death by producing a blood-clotting

enzyme. It is rarely used in supplements, although research has shown it to have great effects in dealing with pain relief and the troubles of old age. Dietary sources include all dark green leafy vegetables, especially cauliflower, cabbage, carrot tops, kale, soya beans, alfalfa, seaweed, pine needles, and fresh seed oils.

- *Calcium* is essential to heart function, and the health and integrity of bones, teeth, blood and nerves. It can be found in dairy produce, but the vegetable world hosts a wide variety of rich sources including kelp, nettles, parsley, chamomile flowers, oats, chicory, dandelion, watercress, seeds and nuts. These are often more easily absorbed than dairy produce. Useful in settling the stomach, and as a buffer when taking vitamin C.
- *Copper* is a component of many chain reactions within the body including the conversion of iron into haemoglobin. Deficiencies are rare, but good dietary sources include shellfish, wheat, dried fruits, almonds and beans.
- *Magnesium* is an antacid that is essential to the growth and repair of cells, promotes healthy function of the glands and regulates the central nervous system. It is involved in over 80 per cent of all activities within the body, and deficiencies are alarmingly common. Good food sources include seafood, nuts, figs, dates, soybeans, cowslips, dandelion, kelp, marshmallow, oats, parsley, raspberries, watercress and spinach.
- *Manganese* works to prevent sterility, keeps the thyroid functioning properly and performs a host of other important functions within the body including regulating blood sugar. It is found in nuts, all dark green leafy vegetables, beetroot, avocadoes, egg yolk, sunflower seeds, pineapple, kelp and whole grains.
- *Phosphorus* works with calcium to maintain bones and

teeth, and is also involved in releasing energy from the cells into a form that we can freely use. Rich sources include wheatgerm, sesame and sunflower seeds, seaweeds, parsley, watercress, dill, liquorice, marigold flowers and leaves, mustard, dandelion leaves, elderberries, nuts and some dairy produce.

- *Potassium* works with sodium in regulating body fluids, and is also needed for proper nerve function. It is to be found in abundance in most herbs and in seaweeds. Other foods containing potassium include: parsley, wheatgerm, dandelion leaves, bananas and apricots.
- *Selenium* protects the individual cells from harm, and overall has an impact on our general resistance to infection. Good sources include seafoods, cereals and wholegrains, nuts and fruit.
- *Sodium* works with potassium in regulating body fluids, and is also involved in all muscle action. Foods that have a perfectly balanced sodium/potassium ratio include: seaweeds, comfrey, dandelion, garlic, fennel, marshmallow, nettles, parsley and watercress.
- *Zinc* is involved in many hormonal actions and affects appetite control and hair growth. Foods rich in zinc include pumpkin and sunflower seeds, brewer's yeast, shellfish, green leafy vegetables and liver. (But please only eat the liver of a humanely reared and killed animal, otherwise the accompanying toxins are horrible.)
- *Iodine* is a component of the thyroid hormones, controlling growth and metabolism. It is found in all produce grown by the sea, because of the iodine-rich soil, and also in seafoods and seaweeds. Seaweed in any form is the best supplement ever of iodine – eat the range for their own tasty properties, or sprinkle some dried over meals, add to baking, etc.

Other substances, usually herbs or spices, can be given in supplement form for ease, or to combine them with effective vitamins or minerals.

Good sources of nutritional supplements include

Lamberts Ltd 1 Lamberts Road, Tunbridge Wells, Kent TN2 3EQ. 01892 552121

Higher Nature Ltd Burwash Common, East Sussex TN19 7LX. 01435 882880

Larkhall Green Farm 225 Putney Bridge Road, London SW5 2PY. 0181 874 1130

Health Plus Ltd Dolphin House, 30 Lushington Road, Eastbourne, East Sussex BN21 4LL. 01323 737374

Recommended reading
The Vitamin Bible Earl Mindell, Vermillion
Off-the-shelf Natural Health Mark Mayell, Boxtree
You Are What You Eat Kirsten Hartvig and Nic Rowley, Piatkus

Tissue Salts

This is a range of minerals in a form that is easily taken and rapidly absorbed by the body. The minerals are shown by their abbreviated Latin names, e.g. Ferr. Phos. (Iron phosphate) and Kali Mur. (potassium chloride). They are formed in tiny lactose tablets and are safe to take for everyone unless there is a lactose intolerance.

Take as directed on the pot and by decanting tablets into the lid and then straight into the mouth, so as not to touch them with the hands. The tablets dissolve very quickly, leaving a slightly sweet taste in the mouth. Effects can often be seen straight away. Their use in practice is often as part of a complex nutritional assessment, but they can also be used very successfully at home for immediate response to specific health concerns. Take them at least 20 minutes away from foods or strong drinks (such as coffee – not that you should be drinking that anyway – or peppermint tea!), or brushing your teeth.

The full range of tissue salts is:

- *Calc. Fluor.* (calcium fluoride) is a greater builder of elastic tissue, and useful for muscular weakness, poor circulation and skin and dental decay.
- *Calc. Phos.* (calcium phosphate) which is vital to the formation of new blood cells, and helps in convalescence and when low in energy.
- *Calc. Sulph.* (calcium sulphate) is a blood purifier that cleanses the skin.
- *Ferr. Phos.* (iron phosphate) increases oxygen carriage by the blood and is particularly useful for older people.
- *Kali Mur.* (potassium chloride) is a blood conditioner and is useful when there is congestion and mucus conditions.
- *Kali Phos.* (potassium phosphate) is a nerve nutrient, invaluable for fretfulness, depression, and nervous headaches.
- *Kali Sulph.* (potassium sulphate) oxygenates the tissue cells, and will show improvements in the skin, hair and nails.
- *Mag. Phos.* (magnesium phosphate) is an antispasmodic and fights cramps, shooting pains and flatulence.
- *Nat. Mur.* (sodium chloride) ensures good water distribution throughout the body and is also useful for runny colds.

- *Nat. Phos.* (sodium phosphate) neutralises acidity, and can help with rheumatic complaints as well as acid indigestion.
- *Nat. Sulph.* (sodium sulphate) eliminates excess water and will help with all congestive complaints from 'flu to water-retention and biliousness.
- *Silica* (silicic oxide) is both cleansing and eliminative and will normalise menstrual cycles as well as helping with bowel function and skin cleansing.

Tissue salts can also be bought as composite remedies to meet different needs:

Combination A for neuralgia and allied conditions
(Combination) B for convalescence and as a general energy booster
C for acidity and heartburn
D for skin complaints
E for flatulence, colic and indigestion
F for nervous headaches and migraines
G for backache and piles
H for hay fever and other allergic responses
I for muscle pain
J for colds, coughs and chestiness (a wonderful seasonal remedy for autumn and winter)
K for brittle nails and hair loss
L for poor circulation
M for rheumatism
N the classic remedy for period pains; also helps with other cramps
P for aching feet and legs
Q for catarrh and sinus complaints
R brilliant for infant's teething pains
S for general nausea, stomach upsets and headaches (the seasonal remedy for summer).

Tissue salts can be bought at healthfood shops, and all good pharmacies.

Recommended reading

A Guide to Biochemic Tissue Salts Dr Andrew Stanway, Van Dyke
The Biochemic Handbook J. S. Goodwin, Thorsons

The Natural World

The elements of earth, air, water and fire form an invaluable part of any healing armoury. Through regular contact with the natural world we reinforce our own health, and we can make contact with each element as magically or as practically as we choose.

The use of air baths and breathing techniques fulfils our need for contact with the air, but so too does going for a walk on a spring morning, and feeling the joy that is in the air along with the varied scents of the emerging flowers. Walking barefoot on grass that is wet with early-morning dew may appeal to the poet within us, but also has marked physical effects that both benefit and strengthen the body. The effects of sunlight on the body are manifold, waking up the pineal gland, stimulating production of vitamin D and melatonin, and reaching in through our skin to warm and comfort the whole body. We can also use the element of fire for its quality of inspiration.

We are made of so much water, it is little wonder that we should have an affinity with this element. Its thermal qualities affect us directly (being used in ice packs, hot and cold packs, compresses, etc.). As a medium for delivering or receiving remedies it is unsurpassed – witness the relief of sinking into a hot bath, or soaking the feet in an Epsom salts footbath at the end of a tiring day.

Water has a wonderfully beneficial effect on the whole system, supplying and suffusing us with soothing negative ions to combat stress. Water can also represent our emotions and be used symbolically to carry away any unwanted feelings.

Following the seasons when it comes to our own health-care makes good all-round sense. Eating foods that are seasonally available keeps our nourishment fresh and meets our need for variety. We can also follow our body's lead and implement health measures that are appropriate to the time of year, like following a fast in spring or autumn, and spending more time in contact with the elements during the warmer months. Often a walk in nature can reinforce our place in the world with all its changes, and this can do a lot to both refresh and de-stress. When we let nature lead, a spring walk can infect us with the enthusiasm, joy and promise that is all around. Summertime lets us bask in the warm energy and ripening of all we see. Autumn brings such a richness as the whole world seems to transform into something that is golden and windswept and embracing change in the fullest sense. The winter landscape can remind us of all that we are nurturing below the ground, in the earth, that great transformer of energies, to be ready to bloom again in springtime.

I am often humbled by taking a walk in the natural world, and it reminds me of my place within it, rather than its place in my life.

Recommended reading
Nature Through the Seasons Richard Adams and Max Hooper, Penguin
Food for Free Richard Mabey, Montana

A Natural Medicine Chest

Many of the items you can use to meet immediate health concerns can be found in your kitchen, or in the garden. Frozen peas make a perfect cold compress for headaches, bruises, and backpain. Vinegar can be added to the bathwater as a regular good health habit for women – it works to normalise the acidity of the vagina and help restore its own self-cleansing ability. It also makes a useful treatment for wasp stings. A mouthful of milk is the only real treatment for a burnt tongue, and bread makes a wonderful poultice to relieve infection.

Plants you can grow in pots on a windowsill, on the patio, or in the garden, and they and their flowers will reward you with their beauty as well as their healing qualities. Useful for healthcare is rose, which makes a wonderful base for pot pourri to scent the house. Simply allow the petals to dry and place in a small pot. Crush whenever you pass, and the gentle scent will be released. Also grow rosemary, thyme, borage and mint for making into teas, adding to inhalations, and to add their vitamins, minerals and delicious flavour to cooking.

Essential oils of Rose, Geranium, Ti-tree, Ylang-ylang, Bergamot and Olibanum are among my most-used favourites. They are unequalled in their flexibility and can be added to bathwater, or compresses for immediate treatment, or used to fragrance a room or clothing.

The range of Flower Remedies is a very individual choice. You may find that you use them for a while and then take a natural break, or that you use just a few for specific situations. From the Bach range, Pine is very useful for weariness, Crab Apple is a good protector when dealing with busy crowds, and Holly is useful for irritation and when seeing people who make you cross. Rescue Remedy is the perfect stand-by for treating burns, cuts, and for dealing with emotional trauma.

Tissue Salts are very useful and can be absorbed directly into the bloodstream to produce immediate benefits. Most people find there are one or two that they are likely to use most often, e.g. Mag. Phos. for period cramps, or Combination B for an instant energy lift. In a family it may be worth keeping the whole range, and these make a particularly good treatment for children.

Taking a multivitamin and mineral supplement is a good idea when stressed, facing health challenges, and at the change of seasons. Individual supplements can be very useful, e.g. vitamin C powder can be added to drinks for instant absorption; it gives an immediate immune boost and makes a natural preservative. Vitamin E capsules can be opened to treat a small burn or to add to any skin preparation. A B-complex supplement is useful for combating stress.

Once you begin to consider using natural remedies, you will be rewarded by their efficacy, ease of use, and most of all by their positive effects on your body.

CHOOSING A PRACTITIONER

Healthcare professionals need to use their care, objectivity, knowledge and experience to interpret your own individual recipe for health, and frame it in a safe and supportive system of practical care. You will need to feel confident and easy with them, and be happy with their ability to communicate and support you in your journey towards full health. This is a very important relationship, and you deserve to make the best possible choice.

Although this is quite different from the system of medicine that forms the basis of our NHS, it is not completely incompatible with it. There are some things that natural healthcare cannot provide, like surgical intervention when the disease process has progressed too far, and we do not have the same financial resources for research and investigative or diagnostic tests. There are, however, many things that we can do better. Within the NHS, 2½ minutes is the average length of a consultation, 92 per cent of medical drugs have side effects, and most multiple prescriptions are for medicines to counteract the effects of other medicines. This is not a recipe for good health.

Time is important in allowing us to talk and recognise our own health history. Spending an hour or more discussing health with a practitioner can bring some real revelations about our approach to our body's needs, and the talking in itself can be very healing.

Natural remedies and methods all work to support the body's own best efforts, and the side effects are all positive and health enhancing. Perhaps most important of all is the holistic approach to health that recognises the unity of our experience, and knows that we cannot divorce the way we think and act from the way we feel both physically and emotionally. Sometimes acknowledging these links is enough to begin a move towards full health.

Visiting any alternative choice of practitioner means paying at the time, as opposed to the pre-payment plan that we have become used to with the NHS. There are of course health insurance schemes to help with costs and many practices have a sliding scale of fees in case of financial difficulty. It makes perfect sense, though, to use the service that you have already paid for, particularly when it can be so useful. I therefore suggest all of my patients have any blood, X-ray or other tests they need done through their GP. I often refer patients back to the GP to confirm a diagnosis, or to pursue a particular course, or even for a prescription – GPs can write up vitamins, minerals and other nutritional supplies, and this is often cheaper than buying them. (They may not always be the most effective, however, as they are likely to be chemically synthesised versions, so follow your practitioner's guidance on this.)

There are many more ways that we could work together to combine what is best about our different approaches and ensure high quality healthcare. Indeed in some areas doctors recommend alternative practitioners, and sometimes work alongside them. Registering with both a Natural Healthcare Practitioner and a GP seems to be the best way to ensure complete care.

I am biased towards Naturopathy as a comprehensive, safe and effective system of healthcare. It starts from the viewpoint that the body is always aiming for optimum health, and seeks many ways to support and encourage this natural intelligence. No naturopathic measures will interfere or intervene with the body's own systems, and they are not invasive in any way. Our view of the whole disease process is that it cannot be fought at the expense of the body – rather that the body can only be reinforced, re-educated and moved towards greater strength, and we seek to reawaken the body's innate ability to slough off any disease states. I say we, because any achievement is always the result of the combined efforts of both patient and practitioner.

This is not always an overnight miracle, and an important aspect of natural healthcare is the relationship between patient and practitioner. When this is encouraging, supporting and enabling, taking the necessary time to address all aspects of concern, then recovery is faster and more lasting. We also need to recognise the integrity of the mind–body–spirit, and know that touching one facet of an individual's experience will impact upon their whole life.

A Natural Healthcare Practitioner is like a natural GP, using a variety of remedies and referrals to ensure the best possible answers to the broad spectrum of health challenges that we all face.

Other complete systems that aim to treat the whole person include Ayurvedic Medicine, Traditional Chinese Medicine, Shamanism, and Cranio-sacral therapy.

Professional Colleges and Associations will be able to give you lists of practitioners in your area, and these will all have completed training in approved courses of study. Beyond that, personal recommendation is a reliable guide.

Further information
The Mandeer Ayurvedic Clinic Hamway Place, London W1.
0171 323 0660

College of Integrated Chinese Medicine, 19 Castle Street, Reading, Berkshire RG1 7SB. 0118 950880
The Faculty of Shamanic Studies PO Box 300, Potters Bar, Hertfordshire EN6 4LE
Karuna (Cranio-Sacral Therapy) Natsworthy Manor, Widecombe-in-the-Moor, Newton Abbot, Devon TQ13 7TR. 01647 221457

GIRLS

Even before the hormonal festival of puberty, girls are notably different to boys. Psychologists and scientists are still exploring their own theories on these differences, but our responses, priorities, psychological make-up, spatial awareness and tastes are all different to boys'. The jury is still out as to what proportions are genetic, acquired or learned.

From the beginning our mothers are our role models for all that we learn how to be. Their beliefs and attitudes will colour our early world with indelible ink. We build throughout our lives on the foundation of their own feelings towards their femininity and what it means to be a woman.

We are influenced by all the expectations of our family and culture. From birth we will be treated differently to boys, but who knows whether things would be different if we were given train sets to play with by people who thought that was completely natural rather than part of the experiment.

Once we arrive at school we will respond strongly to the opportunity for socialisation and relationship, and competition is sometimes harder to learn. According to some psychologists, by that time we will almost certainly have fallen in love with one of our parents, and learned that society likes us to internalise our feelings. (Boys tend to learn how to express themselves more aggressively.) We will probably already be expressing our feelings through our body, but beyond that there is little to distinguish our healthcare needs from those of boys.

Managing Change

Girls growing up from infancy to puberty see tremendous changes. We move out from the security of the family into school, where we develop new friends and relationships. It is often our first opportunity to compare and contrast our own family models with those of others, and can prove to be a challenging time for the whole family. This is also often the time of realising the weight of our parents' expectations for us, and of us, and where we begin to explore structuring our own lives. This is perhaps the first time when we have had our own projects and activities to pursue, independently of the rest of the family.

This can be the beginning of a lifetime of adventure if we have known a secure and loving background. This is the time when mothers have to loosen their ties to their children, and deal with the pain of separation. As girls, of course, we are blissfully unknowing of all the uncomplicated feelings that can surround our coming out into the world.

As guardians of our early life, our parents play a key role in cultivating and fuelling our imagination and sense of self. It is with their assistance, and within the framework that they provide for us, that we can begin to explore what it means to be a true human being. If we are exposed to music, literature, painting, play and exploration, then these elements will be built into our lives. The richness of the care that we receive, and the quality of the time and nourishment that our parents make available to us will form the basis of our ability to love, express tenderness, and experience intimacy in the future. And the model of relationship that our parents express is the one that we will carry with us as a template for our own partnerships.

As children, we are a little like sponges on the emotional and energetic levels, absorbing the atmosphere of our environment as surely as we digest our meals. While parents spell out words, or talk behind closed doors we tend to be able to feel the truth of the situation. One of the best gifts our parents can make to us is to honour our understanding of that truth – to reinforce the validity of our feeling responses. As females in our society we will have the luxury of being able to associate freely with our feelings – it is much more OK for us to cry than it is for boys, and the link between our feelings and our body is more readily accepted.

Another special gift is the introduction to ways of working and manifesting our inner world, through any medium of expression.

Tammy was brought to see me by her mother, after visits to her GP had found no reasons for the tummy pains that had been troubling her. She was a sensitive, rather shy five-year-old, with no other real health concerns, except for the tummy pains that she had experienced quite regularly over the last year.

We agreed that I would give Tammy a physical check-up, and once her mother had left, she and I had the opportunity to have a good chat about her pains, and what was going on in her world. She didn't have any pain at the time, and her structural assessment showed no obvious problems. Her diet was reasonably sound, and her bowel movements were regular and trouble free. She was quite happy at school, and had settled in to her new routine rather well.

Tammy was very protective about her mother, saying again and again what a hard-working, good mother she was to her. I suggested that she must be a great help to her mother, and wondered whether she was like her in many ways. 'We even have a period at the same time' were Tammy's exact words at the end of a long description of how similar she and her mother were, and how she helped her mother shoulder the burden of the family.

Tammy had so wished to express solidarity with her mother, that she was copying her mother's physical responses – she experienced bad cramping with her period, and at ovulation. She never discussed this with her daughter, but when we reviewed the incidents of Tammy's tummy pains they concurred with her mother's dates.

I suggested they both sit down and discuss the periods, and that pain was not a necessary part of them, and also that there be less secrecy around what was happening with the mother's feelings. (We also worked out some health measures to reduce her painful episodes.) Tammy's pains disappeared altogether over the following two weeks, and she and her mother now have a much more open relationship.

Your Body Now

Phenomenal changes occur throughout the body in the years leading up to puberty. It is little wonder then that occasional growing pains appear, but this growing spurt is part of our wonderful design, and no troubles should last for any length of time.

We will by now be fully aware of our parents' pattern of physical activity, and of their expectations of us. Children who come from sedentary households, or homes where physical activity receives a low priority, rarely become sporty types themselves. We follow our parents' example and choose a similar level of activity or inactivity to them. If we can be encouraged to develop our physical side, and explore sporting pursuits, it is a habit that is likely to last us all our lives.

Feeling comfortable with our bodies is also likely to be learned within the family, and specifically from our mothers and the example that they set.

Dancing and movement classes are wonderful exercises for girls, to connect them with their own inner sense of rhythm, and with a style of expression that they may use for their own healing later in life.

One of the most important things for girls to learn is about the changes that are due to happen to their body with puberty. If they feel easy with their physical attributes now, they are more likely to experience a smooth transition into adulthood. Most children have a natural curiosity about their genitalia, and many will have masturbated in some form, usually just putting their hands between their legs and enjoying the feeling, long before puberty. If the subject of sex and the changes they can expect to their body can be handled with sensitivity and care, this can set them up for a lifetime of good feelings and freedom from hang-ups.

If you follow a religion that has negative beliefs about sex and women's bodies, or if you have your own insecurities and hang-ups, you may wish to re-evaluate these before passing them on to your child. Few things are more beautiful than our bodies, and no part of them should be any source of shame or discomfort. I feel it is verging on the criminal to temper a child's innocence with negative, self-deprecating images of themselves and their bodies. If you can make your life easier too by relieving yourself of any such burdens, then so much the better. Investigate counselling to help you sort out your real feelings about this matter, or simply apply some sound common sense, and find ways to change any negative thoughts and feelings that you may be carrying.

What to Eat Now

Feeding a child well is rather like putting money in its constitutional bank. It allows for a degree of depletion in later life without the damage of compromised overall health. The flavours that we are exposed to during childhood colour our preferences throughout life, affecting our tastebuds, and the food choices we are likely to make as we grow older.

Children need to ensure a variety of dietary sources of proteins, fats, carbohydrates, vitamins, minerals and trace elements to ensure adequate building materials for their growing bodies. A diet that is rich in a range of seasonal foods and a variety of nutrient sources encourages a better climate of intestinal bacteria that will influence digestion and assimilation of foods throughout life. These children will also experience the greater sense of physical security that stems from improved constitutional strength, and are less inclined to suffer with minor ailments. They are also either less vulnerable to, or less harmed by, dietary excess and undernourishment in later years.

Children respond extremely quickly to dietary influences. They will often fast spontaneously in order to improve their health or to meet a threatened health difficulty like a cold. Never force children to eat when they really don't have any appetite; let them learn from you that it is good to trust the body and its signals.

Children are notorious for their changing fads and tastes for different foods. If you can be relaxed about this it will pay dividends in their healthy attitude towards nourishing themselves. Similarly, the question of mealtime discipline – to finish what is on the plate or to allow them to eat as much as they feel they need. If your dinner table is friendly, and the atmosphere is relaxed and easy, digestion will be improved and the answer should be fairly easy.

Hyperactivity and other behavioural disorders have been linked to certain foodstuffs. If your child is responding in this way, do consider consulting a natural healthcare practitioner for a full health assessment, but in the meantime avoid all orange food colouring, orange squash, and orange juice. Limit all refined sugar to once a day – that means watching biscuits, sweets, chocolate, cakes, fizzy drinks and squashes. Balance the diet by including whole grains like brown rice and rye, and whole wheat, and drink plenty of water to flush the system. Most people find there is a direct link between the consumption of refined sugars and temper flare-ups, or a definite allergy to orange food colouring.

There is also a link between hyperactivity and a deficiency of Essential Fatty Acids. These can be found in abundance in vegetable oils like sunflower, safflower, wheatgerm and soya, and in green-leaved vegetables. Adding 1,000mg of flaxseed or safflower oil to the diet each day will redress any deficiency. Or you could use it to massage the child's tummy after a bath, and allow it to be absorbed through the skin. This treat can be a relaxing island of calm and quiet, and will enhance your relationship.

Whenever you restrict a child's diet in any way, be careful not to do so for more than one month without professional advice. You may also like to give a child vitamin and mineral supplements at this time, but read the labels carefully to ensure that you are not giving them any of the items that you are avoiding in the diet. The ingredients will all be listed on the box.

Sarah brought her daughter Dominique to me because she was an overactive, fractious five-year-old who couldn't sit still, and became very loud and red faced as she ran around the room shouting every few minutes. She had always been an active child, but things had become much worse since she started at school. Sarah didn't feel Dommy was naughty, but was having to explain things to Dommy's teacher who could not contain her disruptions.

I suggested Sarah keep a diet diary monitoring everything that she gave Dommy, and involve her teacher in noting what she was having at school. I also recommended some regular quiet time at the beginning and end of each day, and after school. I gave Dommy a physical examination using cranial techniques, and that showed no real difficulty, so suggested she remove orange food colouring from their diet altogether and come back to see me again, with the diet diary, in the following week.

At the second appointment, Dommy was able to sit still for at least part of the time. Her diet diary showed a very high intake of sugar, which had doubled since she started school and was swapping sweets with the other children, and of sugary snacks at breaks.

We worked out a diet for her that eliminated refined sugar, and balanced whole grains with suitable snacks for her to take to school. She responded well to dried fruits, and to natural sugars like honey when they were eaten with other, more grounding foods like oats in flapjacks, and rice in ricecakes. We involved her teacher in monitoring her progress at school – they made food a class project and everyone got involved, so Dommy did not feel singled out in any way. Over the next twelve weeks, her behaviour pattern evened out considerably. She still has a strong reservoir of physical and emotional energy, and needs to let off steam regularly, but this has become part of her physical activity, and seems to cause her no distress. Her aptitude and ability to concentrate all improved, and so long as her diet remains controlled, she shows none of the earlier unruly symptoms.

When she has extra sugar, the symptoms tend to reappear, but these can now be more easily managed and understood. When they came back to see me for a six-month review, Dommy sat and played like any other five-year-old.

Staying Well

Follow your own intuition when treating your child, it will usually be right. If you feel uncertain about their condition, or the symptoms seem strange to you, then consult your practitioner. If the child experiences tummy ache which is painful when touched, accompanied by high temperature, seek medical attention. The appendix can cause problems if left unattended when it is inflamed. You will usually be able to distinguish this from regular tummy ache because of the muscle guarding that tends to accompany it.

Bedwetting

This can be helped by warming and supporting the kidneys, and also by addressing any fears in the child's life. One cup every other day of parsley or yarrow tea will begin to support and strengthen kidney function. Place ¼ teaspoon of the dried herb in boiling water for ten seconds, then remove, and sip slowly while still warm. One cup of St John's Wort tea can be tried instead, to life the spirits and ease any concerns. Make in the same way, and try for about one week, before switching to other measures.

Add one drop each of Dr Bach's Crab Apple and Rescue Remedy to a little almond or olive oil, and use this to massage the kidney area once a week. Make this quite a stimulating, warming massage, stroking out from the spine with both hands, and circling the whole kidney region repeatedly.

Reduce or eliminate salt in the diet, and make sure no drinks are taken after supper. Give the tissue salt Nat. Mur. in the dose described on the tub on the day after each episode, or at a maximum dose for three days each week. The fine cornsilk that is revealed when corn on the cob is uncovered is a good tonic for this region, and a little can be eaten each day, or made into a weak tea and taken before meals.

It is important not to make too much fuss about these measures, and that the child is not blamed or punished in any way for bedwetting. Sometimes children will wet themselves during the day too. If this is the case, it is wise to discuss this with the child and check that any worries or concerns they may have are being dealt with. Check, too, that they know the sensations of a full bladder. (Pelvic floor exercises may help, see p.175).

Coughs, colds and 'flu

Children can be prone to all sorts of colds and sniffles. If persistent mucus conditions are a problem, tackle the diet first. Remove mucus-forming foods as much as possible (dairy products, wheat, refined sugar and red meat), and increase the amount of fresh vegetables, garlic and ginger root. Avoid eating anything frozen, like ice-cream, or food straight from the 'fridge. Add a little turmeric to the diet – this Indian spice is very effective for removing phlegm. Sprinkle a pinch onto cooked meals, use to flavour oils or add to rice near the end of cooking time.

Red sage is the herb of choice for all sore throats and minor coughs. Make a weak infusion by steeping ¼ teaspoon of the dried herb in a mug of boiling water for thirty seconds. Half of this is to be drunk, and ideally the child would gargle with the other half. If this is not possible, use to wash the mouth out, and make a throat pack with the remaining liquid. Take a thin strip of cotton fabric that is long enough to wrap once around the neck, and steep it in the remaining infusion. Wring out well, and apply to the neck, covering it with a thin towel or similar wrapping to both hold it in place and protect the rest of the body. This can be worn to bed and left on through the night.

To keep the chest clear, spread a dab of oil on the ball of the foot and place a peeled clove of garlic there, holding it in place throughout the night by wrapping in a sock. If the chest is troubled, wrap the child in a chest pack (see p.56), put to bed and check on them through the night.

Do not feed the child, the appetite will often be suppressed anyway. Make sure there is lots to drink, including fresh vegetable juices and give a weak infusion of peppermint tea once a day. If possible, give a children's chewable vitamin C tablet at least once each day with a drink or snack.

If the child becomes sticky and uncomfortably warm in bed, sponge down with a tepid infusion of lime flowers or thyme. Make a teapot full of the infusion using one–two teaspoons of the dried herbs, steep for three minutes, then strain into a large bowl of warm water, and cool to a comfortable temperature before applying.

Place a drop of Olbas oil or Eucalyptus essential oil on the pillow, and add one drop of Thyme essential oil to a burner in the room, or add to a cup of boiled water placed near the bed. These will all work to clear the nose and chest and make breathing easier.

Ear- and toothache

In both cases, limit the diet to warm drinks and fresh vegetable juices if desired. For ears, add one drop of warmed almond oil to the outside cavity of each ear, and stop with a little cotton wool plug that has been dipped into the warm oil. Apply an onion poultice to the back of the neck overnight to draw out any local impurities. This may also be used for toothache. Spread a dab of oil on the back of the neck, and cover with the poultice, which can be wrapped or held in place with a tea towel or strip of cotton fabric tied like a scarf around the neck. Make the poultice very simply by grating ¼ of a fresh onion on to a thin cotton bandage and applying straight away.

For toothache, apply a little oil of cloves to the gum and around the tooth. Massage the outside of the cheek with a little ghee, and if the pain is severe add one drop of Dr Bach's Rescue Remedy.

Hopi Ear Candles are remarkably effective for cleansing and healing this whole area. You can get them from your local healthfood shop and follow the directions, or ask your practitioner to perform the procedure for you.

Fears

Expressing fears and panics is a 'normal' part of childhood. They are an exciting and exhilarating adventure that can link children together. Fashions can change from week to week, or more appropriately from one school term to another, often spreading quickly through the playground.

Whether it is screams at spiders, or panics about unseen threats such as the bogey man, these can often be regarded as transitional, and a healthy way of letting off steam. Only if behaviour becomes worrisome, or if the child appears withdrawn or disturbed by events, should there be any real cause for concern.

A number of Dr Bach's Flower Remedies are aimed specifically towards combating fears.

- Rock Rose is a good emergency remedy for dealing with shock or panic.
- Mimulus works with quiet, cold fears that include being alone, and worry over situations or events that could occur in reality.
- Cherry Plum is the remedy for guilt and concern over one's own actions.
- Aspen is for vague, unknown, unspeakable fears.
- Red Chestnut for those over-concerned about other's worries.

Use three drops of any combination of the above remedies and apply to the pulse points on the temple, neck, wrists and behind the knees. This can be repeated three times a day.

Another method is to add some of the mixture to a little warm water, and soak the hands or feet in this for five minutes before bed.

A cup of dilute infusion of Heartsease may be taken once a day. Prepare by pouring boiling water onto ½ teaspoon (2.5ml) of the dried herb. Steep for thirty seconds and drink while still warm.

Counselling can be tremendously useful if there is no response to the above measures. Often a single chat with an experienced and friendly professional can be enough to set improvements in motion.

Headaches and general malaise

It is not uncommon for children to have occasional days when they simply need to rest. When you consider all the growth and change that their body and awareness is embracing, it is little wonder that there is sometimes a need to stop and renew. Check that there is no regular pattern to any sickness, such as games day at school, or the visit of a particular relative. If you discover this is the cause, discussing it in a sensitive way may uncover the root of any difficulty.

Put the child to bed and place a cool compress on their forehead and on the back of the neck. Make this by soaking a thin strip of cotton fabric in a linden flower tissane that has been kept in the fridge. Wring out well and apply, changing it as soon as it becomes warm. This soothing application will often encourage rest, if not sleep. Minimise foods for the day, and give plenty of fresh diluted juices to drink. Rose petal tea is a wonderful soother, and can be made easily from the roses in the garden so long as they have not been treated with chemicals. Cram a teapot full of the rose petals and cover with boiling water. Allow to steep for five–ten minutes, before pouring out, and drink when tepid or cool, having added a little honey and a fresh rose petal to the cup.

Nits and worms

These occur in the healthiest of households and to the cleanest of families. Any remaining stigma attached to these sorts of troubles is not based on fact. Use a walnut leaf wash (see below) massaged into the scalp each day for three–five days to remove lice. If there is no response, switch to a combination of one tablespoon of clear, white alcohol (vodka is good) with five drops of Thyme essential oil and two tablespoons (28ml) of sesame oil. Rub into the hair and scalp and leave in overnight. Wash well the next morning, and rinse with a dilute infusion of rosemary. It is advisable for the whole family to do this, and for all bedding, cushions that may have been lain upon, and towels to be well washed. Make sure to clean hairbrushes, ties, etc., too.

To clear thread or tape worms from the system, give the child fifteen–twenty raw pumpkin seeds and ensure they are chewed very well (you can make this into a game by seeing how long each seed can stay in the mouth, or how many chews it will survive). If this is not possible, they can be pounded into a fine gruel, mixed with water and spoonfed. After thirty minutes, give one teaspoon (5ml) of castor oil. Ensure that the diet is rich in fresh garlic and ginger root for the next three days. Again, it is a good idea for the whole family to take the cure. It can be repeated every three days while there is a suspicion of worms.

Roundworms can be eliminated by taking two peeled onions, two peeled garlic cloves, and a one-inch (2cm) long piece of peeled horseradish root. Add to one pint (570ml) of milk in a saucepan, and boil for three minutes. Allow to cool to drinking temperature, and sip until it is all gone. This tastes filthy, but does the trick, acting very quickly. The hotter it is when drunk, the less 'flavoursome' the drink.

Scabies can be effectively treated by bathing the affected areas with a walnut leaf wash, or the freshly juiced stems of calendula plants. To make the wash, add two tablespoons (28ml) of finely chopped walnut leaves to one pint (570ml) of hot water. Steep for thirty seconds, then strain off the liquid. Apply once it is cool enough to handle.

Travel sickness

Motion sickness is not uncommon in children. Simple measures such as ensuring a good source of fresh air, and scheduling plenty of stops for the child to just sit and be still, will often cure the problem. Otherwise, give a small piece of crystallised ginger to chew one hour before travelling, and every thirty minutes throughout the journey. You may also purchase a 'travel band' from the chemist. This is a simple sweat band that is worn around the wrist. Sewn into the fabric is a plastic bead that will press onto the acupuncture point that helps settle nausea.

Mumps, measles, etc.

These diseases of childhood are a good opportunity for the body to rid itself of toxins that have built up in the system, although if the mother's constitution is strong and the pregnancy was untroubled, then the growing child may not need these health crises to do this. When they do occur, encourage elimination through all the body systems, consider applying a body pack (see below) and give lots of water to drink to help sweating and bowel movements. Consult your practitioner for individual care and advice regarding the pros and cons of inoculations.

Body and chest packs

To make a chest pack, wring out a clean cotton handkerchief in cold water, and put this directly on the child's chest. Cover immediately with a towel, then wrap the child up in a sheet and blankets or a quilt. Make sure that the child is well covered, up to the chin. The child will usually warm up very quickly, and the combination of moist warmth and the comfort of the wrapping ensures a good night's sleep. Do this just before bedtime and leave the pack in place overnight, checking the child at least once by placing a hand inside the layers of wrapping: the handkerchief should be warm and drying.

To make a body pack for a child, use two handkerchiefs or tea towels, and lie the child on one, placing the other on the chest so that most of the upper body is sandwiched between the wet cloths. Wrap up well as before, and check during the night.

These can also be used by adults, for whom it may be easier to slip on a cold, wet cotton vest and layer up with a cotton T-shirt and jumper before wrapping up in a quilt or blankets.

Resources

Kitty Campion's Handbook of Herbal Health Kitty Campion, Sphere

The Massage Book George Dawning, Penguin

A Parent's Guide to Complementary Healthcare for Children Pippa Duncan, Newleaf

Women's Health Information Centre 52 Featherstone Street, London EC1Y 8RT. 0171 251 6580

Women's Health and Reproductive Rights Information Centre 52–4 Featherstone Street, London EC1Y 8RT. 0171 251 6580

British Association for Counselling 1 Reget Place, Rugby CV21 2PJ. 01788 550899

National Council of Psychotherapists and Hypnotherapy Stream Cottage, 98 Wish Hill, Willingdon, East Sussex BM20 9HQ. 01323 501540

PUBERTY

Puberty is marked by immense physical and inner changes and it culminates in the flow of the first menstrual period, at about eleven to fifteen years of age. It is a preparation for the onset of a continuous cycle of change that will last for the next twenty-five to forty years. Within a relatively short timespan, breasts begin to develop, there are obvious changes in the skin and circulation, and the appearance of pubic hair and fat stores considerably changes the overall appearance and shape of a girl's body.

Hormones are responsible for these inner changes, and for many of the emotional and feeling responses that accompany them.

Puberty sees the flowering of our own individuality through the haze of enormous hormonal, societal and often family pressures. It is now that the foundations of healthy attitudes towards the body, menstruation, and sex receive their first proving. Self-esteem and emotional stability are all heavily challenged, and there can seem to be no constancy at all amidst the constant flood and flux of physical and emotional feelings, desires and changes.

This may also be a wonderfully rich time in life, when we are almost literally 'busting out all over' – full of expectation and promise, with boundless energy, and discovering and effecting change and adventure at every turn. Usually adolescence encompasses all of these experiences, in rapid succession.

This is commonly the first occasion when we will be perceived as women and experience the world from a new gender-based identity. Accompanying this emerging femininity come potential worries from peer pressures and altered family relationships. Monumental inner change is occurring too, with the appearance of the first menstrual period, the development of breasts and body hair, and an often confusing sexual appetite. Concerns about acne, menstrual regularity and bra sizes can make for a turbulent and potentially difficult transition into adult womanhood. It can sometimes feel as though we are terribly alone, and bucking a world of difference, at a time when we are least equipped to do so.

Managing Change

Separating our external and internal worlds can be a daunting prospect, yet recognising where the roots of our experience sit can yield tremendous benefits, especially during times of transition. Realising that we each have a part of us that needs to belong, alongside a very real desire to kick out on our own, lays the seed for an appreciation of paradox that can act as a guide throughout life. It can help make sense of difficult and changing relationships at home and school, and shed some light on rebelliousness, and handling peer pressures.

It is OK to want more than one thing at any one time, or to feel drawn in more than one direction. The key to managing this successfully lies in granting yourself permission to have a whole variety of different views, opinions, wants, desires and needs – all at the same time. Not needing to suppress or hide any of these allows you to then make some choices about which to pursue and develop, which to keep private and to yourself, and which to drop for now.

Making your own decisions about matters that directly impact on your life is an important adult skill. The principles developed now may remain with you throughout your life, or be changed, altered or abandoned, the choice is yours. Until now it was parents and teachers, elders, society's views, Church teachings, and advertising that informed your world. It can be daunting and a little frightening to take on that power for ourselves, yet it doesn't mean that we can't still receive support, encouragement, guidance and teachings from a whole variety of sources – just that the choice is now our own.

The inner changes experienced at this time may lead to a desire for experience and experimentation with all that is new and has so far been unavailable. There is a very real need to separate from our parents and to live differently to them, and the status quo of family life can be shattered by challenges to parental authority. That relationships are capable of altering beyond recognition can sometimes be a good thing.

The expressiveness of the father–daughter bond often changes as the girl child suddenly becomes a potentially sexual, menstruating woman, and there can be undercurrents of rivalry and jealousy as the mother's position as the woman of the house is challenged. Riding these changes requires openness and communication by all family members. Celebrating the changes as they occur, and acknowledging the shifting roles and responsibility can transform this into a time of strengthened family unity and love.

We all have our own subjective concept of reality. Most of us find great similarity with the existing paradigm and achieve conformity to a large degree. Our inner worlds, kept private in the most part, allow the richness of our own unique vision to surface. Now is the time to begin to foster those inner truths, and keeping a dream diary is a wonderful way to start.

KEEPING A DREAM DIARY

This is a lovely way to honour your dreams, and can prove a valuable guide to an emerging inner world. It can prove a strong anchor to have such a focus, and the simple act of making each diary entry will help clarify the messages that are coming into your awareness through the dreams. The revelations that can arise from studying our quieter desires and motivations make useful guides in everyday reality.

Begin by choosing a book in which to make your daily record. This can be any notepad, it doesn't have to be special in any way other than you choose, so you might like to decorate it yourself, or have a special colour for the cover. Then choose a pen or pencils, and keep these by your bed ready to write in as soon as you wake.

The next step is to think about recording and remembering your dreams, and spend a few days getting used to the idea.

Before sleeping, then, on the next night, ask to remember your dreams. Let this be your last thought as you go to sleep, and write down whatever you can as soon as you wake the next day.

Your commitment to the process is to write down what you remember having experienced during the night. It doesn't matter if that is 'I don't remember anything' for the first few nights, or a mixture of seemingly dissociated images. Some entries might be drawings of images that you have woken up with filling your mind. Or you might like to write on only one side of the page, and leave the other side free for a diary insert that shows what was happening in your waking or emotional world. Stick with your commitment, and you will see a whole new world begin to unfold. One of the joys of keeping a journal in this way is that you can go back and look at any recurrent themes that your dreams may have, or chart the changing images that appear over time.

Your Body Now

Puberty is a time of great inner and outer change. Beyond the spurts of growth that marked childhood, now the physical changes almost all signal an emerging woman.

There are many ways to strengthen and support that nascent femininity. It is important to realise that each of us is growing and blossoming to our own individual recipe. Breasts, periods and the rest all appear when they will, without regard to friends, expectations, or even the laws of symmetry. The most powerful way to influence this process is with a positive self-image that greets each new event and finds pleasure and satisfaction in this wonderful emerging womanhood.

Accessory physical changes are occurring all over the body. As breasts grow and weigh on the chest wall, so there is a tendency to become round shouldered. This is especially so because in our culture, pert, upturned breasts are a signal of sexual readiness. Many young girls who do not feel ready for such encounters feel they can hide their breasts by stooping. Actually, the sight of a young girl unnaturally hunched over is far more eyecatching. A well-fitting bra will both minimise the effect and provide comfortable support. Those whose breasts develop more slowly can also encounter postural difficulties in their efforts to make the chest stand out. Add to this the structural pressures placed by wearing high heels and carrying shoulder bags, and the body can often need a little re-educating.

Alternate heel height as much as possible, and, if carrying

anything heavy, wear the strap across the body rather than just on one shoulder or the other. Once a day, every day, do the following exercise to remove any kinks, and maintain flexibility and suppleness in the spine.

WALL SLIDE EXERCISE

Stand with your back against a wall, placing your feet together and your heels back up against the skirting. Press your spine back against the wall and take a few deep breaths. Feel your body 'give' a little as it relaxes and accepts the strong support of the wall. Let your chin drop slightly so that your neck is relaxed and you are looking straight ahead. Feel your arms lengthen slightly as they hang freely by your side.

Just for reference, take one hand to the small of your back and feel any gap between it and the wall, then return it to your side.

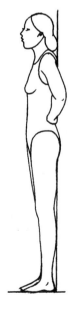 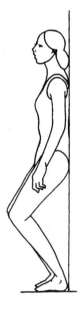

Keeping your knees together as much as you can, and your feet flat on the floor, slowly slide down the wall as far as you can comfortably go. Your pelvis will automatically be tilting forward slightly, and reducing any gap between your lower back and the wall. You can increase this by tightening your lower abdominal muscles. When you have reached the limit of your slide, hold that position while you take a few deep breaths. Then see if you can drop just a little further, feeling stretches in your leg muscles as well as in your lower back.

Slowly straighten up, release your abdominal muscles and uncurl your pelvis.

Repeat this three to five times, keeping the movements of each slide fluid and resisting any urge to bounce.

Amanda was a likeable teenage girl, tall for her age and very sporty. Her mother brought her to see me because of back pain that seemed to get worse as she sat for long periods of time, both in class and when doing homework.

A physical assessment showed some early postural difficulty that responded well to cranial treatment. After the first session, Mandy reported a 50 per cent improvement – she was able to sit still for longer than before, and the pain was not so bad as it had been. She stopped carrying her heavy school bag over her shoulder, and was careful to maintain good posture. We also looked at the ergonomics of her working position – ensuring that she was sitting at the right height for the desk, and relaxing her lower back by propping her feet up on a footstool or small pile of books.

We raised her working surface very simply, but letting her write on top of a couple of books at school, and getting her a new desk at home. She had six further treatments of cranial work, and continued to do some remedial exercises to strengthen her back. At her annual check-up she was doing just fine, and the back pain had not recurred.

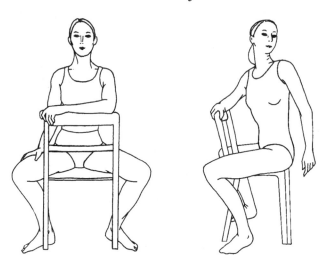

CHAIR TWIST EXERCISE

Sit astride an upright chair facing forwards with your feet flat on the floor. Place your right forearm along the top of the chairback, and grip the end with your hand. Use this hold to gently and slowly pull your upper body round to the left as far as you can comfortably go. Turn your head to the left and take a few deep, relaxing breaths, letting go of any tension. Then see if you can ease yourself round just a little bit further, taking care not to make any jerky movements. Slowly return to the forward-facing position and change arms. Lay your left forearm along the top of the chairback, ready to gently and slowly pull your upper body round to the right. At full stretch turn your head to the right and take a few deep, relaxing breaths. See if you can stretch your body just a little further, then return to the front.

Make all these movements fluid and smooth, and resist any urge to jerk. Repeat the complete movement three times.

What to Eat Now

Difficulties ranging from depression and acne to sinusitis may appear during puberty. Good dietary and exercise habits will help considerably at this time, as will a willingness to support and enhance the body's own efforts to effect good, healthy changes.

A well-balanced diet that emphasises fresh food and includes at least five servings of fruit and vegetables a day will build good foundations. Avoiding junk food and too many snack meals and confectioneries will help maintain energy levels and avoid bad habits. Drink plenty of water, diluted fruit and vegetable juices and herbal teas in place of sugared, carbonated drinks, and keep stimulants such as coffee and alcohol to a minimum.

It is important to gain a good understanding of nutrient values and to explore, for example, alternative sources of protein, and food combinations that will ensure a full range of nutrients with each meal. Vegetarians also need to ensure a full range of B-vitamins in their diet.

This is a time when our bodies grow, change shape, and become obviously feminine. There can be any number of reasons for wanting to check this, including issues around loss of control, and fears of what it means to be a woman in our society. One way to control our development directly is through the way we eat.

Our own sense of the feminine is gained in large part from our mothers, and from women in the family, and also from what we see in the outside world. In a society that is not very welcoming to women, we can be tempted not to want to join! This is also the first time that we can take over responsibility for feeding and nurturing ourselves. Until now, this has been the domain of the mother or other prime carer.

Eating disorders are common in our society, yet like many other women's ailments, we can feel as though we are suffering entirely alone. This is commonly an age of experimenting with diets and lifestyle changes, and the discipline of regular mealtimes can easily go by the board. It can sometimes be hard to tell whether there is any real problem with eating, and it is often difficult to admit to, even to oneself. Difficulties such as binge eating, not eating, or eating and then making yourself sick, are all signs of unhappiness or tensions that have little to do with food, and lots to do with feelings. Sometimes feelings and emotions can feel so uncomfortable that we just want the pain or the chaos to stop, and when we can't make that happen, we control what we can in our life.

Some food-related difficulties just resolve themselves as we grow more accustomed to life and our emotional responses. At other times they can grow until they become much more noticeable and impact on the whole family and other areas of life.

There is a range of different therapeutic options that can all prove helpful, from family therapy to physical support with herbs. Sometimes the healing is in the journey through these different practices, or in finding the right balance of different measures. In all cases, the counselling and support of an experienced practitioner is essential to ultimate success.

How, when and what we eat, therefore, is a topic that can contain much power, and many emotional undertones. When and how we eat is every bit as important as the substances we consume. Bodies need a regular intake of suitable energy to meet our varied daily needs, and sticking to a routine of regular mealtimes is the best way to ensure this. The digestive fire within the body, just like the sun, is at its peak at noon. This is traditionally the time for the largest meal of the day, and food eaten in the middle of the day is more quickly absorbed and metabolised.

Digesting food requires energy. It is a complex process that involves many small yet important stages in order to obtain the maximum nutritional content from each meal. You can respect your body's inner processes by giving yourself a calm environment, and, most important, stillness when eating. Enhance your enjoyment and your nourishment by sharing mealtimes with others who embrace these ideals. When you are happy and feel good, all your digestive processes are improved, so have fun and be good to your body.

This is a time of questioning moral values amongst many other things, and, as part of this, alternative ways of eating can prove attractive, especially as they can seem to offer a fast fix for certain ills. Sometimes other cultures can offer an exciting mealtime alternative to the familiar fare of earlier years. As food is a strong power tool, the dinner table can become something of a battleground. Suspect areas are most definitely animals and their derivatives, and mealtimes offer an obvious occasion for debate. While raising animals for food is certainly a moral question, ethics aside there can be little doubt of the health risks in eating food that is heavily adulterated with the cocktail of chemicals, hormones and antibiotics used in many modern livestock farming methods. But eating the flesh of animals who have known only hardship and fear also means taking that energy into your body. Make yourself aware of the possibilities for keeping animals in a way that maintains both their dignity and our own, and to ensure them an honourable death. More humanely managed sources of animal products are becoming available, and this makes for more of a choice in this area.

If considering making major changes to the diet, like becoming vegetarian, vegan, or losing weight, be sure to take good advice first to ensure that the basic diet remains as nutritious and health-enhancing as it needs to at this key time. It is not sufficient to eliminate a major food group; good nutritious substitutes need to be identified and included on a permanent basis.

I had treated Harriet in the past, and she brought her daughter Jane to see me because of general worries about the girl's health. She was fifteen and was having a hard time, being considered at school and at home as rather 'difficult'. She had occasional temper bursts, but was most often sullen and lifeless, spending lots of time alone in her room doing nothing very much, and always seemed to be troubled with colds and a runny nose.

Jane seemed disinterested, and slightly resentful at being brought to see me, but we soon managed to find some common ground when I asked about what motivated her. She was passionate about animal rights, and felt very frustrated that she could not yet be active in effecting any change in the world. She felt rather powerless and stifled, believing that her mother would not understand, and had not even told her that she was now totally vegetarian.

Jane had been simply avoiding the meat in meals at home, and doubling up on cheese on toast, and other snacks. Her particular favourites were risotto, pizza, and spaghetti. When we removed cheese from her diet her cold symptoms disappeared, and cutting down on wheat meant her energy levels bounced up again. Discussing the matter with her mother, she found that Harriet was also committed to improving animal welfare, and together they managed to both restructure the family meals to include less meat and incorporate good protein sources for Jane, and also to plan ways of educating other local families and friends about animal welfare.

When Harriet came to see me three months later, she said things had never been better at home, and Jane was brighter, happier and much more active. She was now able to include dairy foods in her diet so long as she did not overdo it, and they had both just returned from a weekend course on vegetarian cooking.

Staying Well

• Changing hormone levels alter the skin's rate of secretion and perspiration. This makes personal hygiene of key importance. Daily dry skin brushing with a natural bristle brush will improve the skin's eliminative ability, remove any risk of blockage causing spots, and enhance overall health. For illustration, see over.

SKIN-BRUSHING

Use a natural bristle brush and brush your skin all over before bathing for best results. Start with a gentle pressure, and build up to a firm brushing stroke that stimulates and invigorates your whole body. Begin brushing the soles of your feet and then brush up both legs. Carry on up the back and front of the torso, going gently over the breasts. Brush up each arm from the fingers, and then down the neck and across the shoulder area. (See illustration, page 72.) You can brush the head, but it is best to avoid the delicate skin on the face.

If skin-brushing regularly, the need for soap and other applications is considerably reduced. Most people find they need to use much less deodorant, if any.

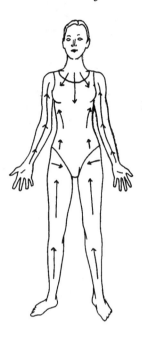

- A good alternative to talcum powder is to mix a dried, powdered herb in equal parts with fuller's earth. This can be used to fill an empty talcum powder shaker. Add elder leaves or mugwort and sprinkle in shoes to help aching feet and check excessive perspiration. Add rose petals for a wonderfully fragrant all-over application, and marigold flowers to soothe troubled skin.
- Commercial skincare preparations can be hard on young skin. To make a good herbal cleanser for oily skin, combine equal parts of buttermilk with a strong infusion of Lady's mantle and store in the fridge. To make the infusion pour ¼ pint (150ml) of boiling water over two tablespoons (28ml) of Lady's mantle leaves and leave to cool. Strain into the buttermilk and use as needed.
- After cleansing, a herbal toner can be used for its astringent qualities. This needs to be made up daily to retain the

active properties of the herbs. Make an infusion by steeping one tablespoon (15ml) of dried sage, marigold or violet leaves, or elderflowers. Leave to stand and use as soon as it is cooled to refresh the skin and remove any traces of cleanser or soap.

Managing stress

Stress can affect us at all stages in life, it is not limited to corporate types reaching mid-life crises. The pressures of exams, unresolved family tensions, and all the other challenges that teenagers face cause their own very real stresses. While some pressures motivate and inspire us, others can feel just too much. It is important to know some good coping mechanisms while we are busy learning which is which.

A first step is to learn some relaxed breathing. This is a simple technique that can form the basis of many different relaxations and can be used instantly whenever the situation requires it.

Start by sitting comfortably with your feet flat on the floor, or you can do this lying down with a pillow under your knees to keep your lower back relaxed. Place your left hand flat on your upper chest, quite close to your collarbone. Place your right hand on your belly, close to your belly button. Now you just need to breathe and see what happens. Most often, you will be able to see your left hand rising and falling, perhaps significantly, with each breath.

Relaxed breathing requires you to allow your breathing to 'drop' down into your belly, and you can begin this by relaxing your chest and shoulders, and imagine each new intake of fresh air being funnelled down to meet your right hand. Practise making your right hand move gently up and down, or in and out, as your lower chest expands with each breath. Your left hand will remain still.

Once you get used to this way of breathing you will find yourself using it more and more often, but initially practise for about ten minutes each day, and start using it if you feel yourself to be in a stressful or pressurised situation.

Acne

Changes in the skin during puberty may lead to 'teenage acne'. This primarily affects the face, chest, upper arms and back, although it may appear in other areas of the body. This is caused when the skin increases its functions of producing both perspiration and sebum, a necessary oil.

Acne occurs when sebum production exceeds the body's other growth functions, e.g. when the rate of growth of new skin cells lags behind, and pores become blocked allowing inflammation and infection to occur.

Good skincare is essential, so use a gentle cleanser daily, and don't be tempted to squeeze the spots. Use a facial steamer at least once a week, or do this the old-fashioned way by pouring boiled water into a large bowl and covering it with a towel to retain the steam. Put your head in under the towel and breathe in the warm steam. Add sprigs of rosemary or thyme to the water for their astringent and antiseptic qualities. If the spots are painful, cut open a leek and paint the juice on before bed. Leave this on overnight and cleanse your skin as normal the next morning. Do not be tempted to dry the skin with strong 'anti-oil' medications. At this stage, the skin is likely to produce extra oil to redress any perceived lack.

Add plenty of raw and cooked cabbage to the diet to cleanse the skin from the inside, and drink plenty of water. Take one cup of nettle tea every day. Make this by steeping one teaspoon of dried nettle leaves in hot water for thirty seconds, and sipping the tea while it is still hot. In the spring, cut the tops of young, clean nettle plants and eat once a week as a vegetable or made into a soup.

Peer pressure

The best answer to anybody who is pressuring you with their own conceptions of what is right, or of what is wrong, with you, is the simple quote: 'Your opinion of me is none of my business'. Whatever other people's convictions, beliefs or prejudices, it is what you know to be true, and best for yourself, that is important. This knowing will often be supported by family, elders, or others close to you, and one of the opportunities of this stage in life is to develop a strong sense of who you are, what you want, and how best you can manifest that.

It is worth remembering that most people of this age are going through similar difficulties, and that what makes others seem so different is only that they use other ways to deal with things. Some push out their anger and appear aggressive, others keep quiet and may appear cool simply because they do not know what to say. Everybody is experiencing the transition and finding their own way to deal with it.

Depression

Feelings of depression often stem from suppressed anger. When we put most of our energy into stopping something, there is little left over to animate, inspire or motivate us. As a society we have many embargoes against the expression of feelings, and anger is perhaps the most unacceptable. Sitting on it, then, is quite a natural thing to do, especially during times of great change and uncertainty.

Anger is an energy, just like everything else. It is only when it festers and ferments that it becomes unpalatable, or when it is accompanied by violent action. These pairings are not fixed, however, and it is perfectly possible to express anger in a million safe, spontaneous ways. The key is in the expression.

Physical activity is a good way to release any pent-up feelings. This can be directed into any number of pursuits, from a strenuous run to an hour of wild dancing, or some vigorous house-cleaning. It is amazing how much energy can be found by even the most lethargic individual once a release is initiated.

This is very much an age of experimenting and discovering our own inner landscape. Melancholy, hopelessness and depression are as important a part of our palette of emotions as are joy, exuberance and pleasure. Short sojourns in any of the 'darker' emotions are quite natural and encourage self-understanding. It is only if those feelings linger that they can become problematic. Doing something about it is often the best form of therapy, and adding uplifting essential oils to the bath (Geranium and Olibanum are good to try), or taking a mix of Dr Bach's Flower Remedies twice a day are good places to start.

Place a flowering jasmine plant on the windowsill to allow the uplifting fragrance to work its effects throughout the day, and eat half a pomegranate, or take one glass of pomegranate juice, every day to raise the spirits.

If the problem persists, check for food intolerance (by eliminating suspect food(s) for a period of time on an exclusion diet), and consider consulting a professional counsellor who has experience of this type of complaint. The idea of having an allergy to foods we eat often can still be a bit of a surprise, but symptoms such as headaches, tiredness, irritability and susceptibility to colds and 'flu can all be traced to foods we eat every day. Our response to foods is uniquely our own, and people respond differently in their allergic response too – I once knew a girl who fainted whenever she ate any vinegar.

Wheat and cows' dairy produce are two of the greatest suspects in terms of food allergy, having an irritating effect on most people. An amazing number of people will find that they have, perhaps, toast for breakfast, a roll or biscuit mid-morning, a sandwich for lunch, a small bun or cake at tea-time, and pasta for dinner. That is a pretty constant everyday intake of wheat. Cows' dairy produce can appear throughout the diet too. Milk on cereal, in tea and coffee, and as a base for milk-shakes, custards, cream toppings and cheeses, in white sauce and in enriched doughs, as a thickener in many pre-cooked meals and as the basis for many ice-creams and other desserts.

Check for these large food groups if looking for potential allergens, and consider also vinegar-based and other acid foods such as tomatoes, spicy foods, peppers, alcohol and red meat.

Resources
Better Health through Natural Healing Ross Trattler, Thorsons
Women's Bodies, Women's Wisdom Dr Christine Northrup, Piatkus
Dieting Makes You Fat Geoffrey Cannon and Hetty Einzig, Sphere
The New Beauty Michelle Dominique Leigh, Newleaf
The Vegetarian Society Parkdale, Dunham Road, Altrincham, Cheshire WA14 4QG. 0161 928 0793
The Soil Association 86/88 Colston Street, Bristol BS1 5BB. 0117 929 0661
Compassion in World Farming Charles House, 5A Charles Street, Petersfield, Hampshire GU32 3EH. 01730 264208

MENSTRUATION

The wonder of the first period heralds a sometimes hesitant beginning to the next thirty to forty years of monthly bleeding. This is one of the great mysteries of the feminine experience. The period is a natural clock that reminds us of our cyclic nature, and offers us the opportunity to review the events of the previous month, and to rest and replenish ourselves. As women who can be continually giving of care and energy, menstruation is a natural time to recharge and rejuvenate; to take a rest from nurturing others and find nourishment for ourselves. This is one of the main events that connects us with all other women, throughout time – imagine, this experience connects Cleopatra, Mary Magdalene, Boadicea, Elizabeth I, Jeanne d'Arc and you!

Each monthly cycle is governed by the action of a variety of hormones. The co-ordinator of all this hormonal activity is the pituitary gland, situated in the brain, close to an area called the hypothalamus.

The hypothalamus influences emotion, weight, sleep, appetite, and water balance. It is affected by other areas of the brain concerned with the senses, thought, memory and creativity. Through understanding how these mechanisms interact, we can piece together some seemingly disassociated aspects of our menstrual cycle. Symptoms such as Pre-Menstrual Syndrome and water retention (see pp.98 and 99) suddenly seem to make sense in terms of what is happening with our hormones.

Each cycle follows an average twenty-nine day course, although it may be as short as eighteen days, or as long as thirty-six, and bleeding usually lasts around five days.

At the beginning of each cycle, the hypothalamus sends signals to the pituitary gland. This instigates the production of two hormones which will govern the first half of the menstrual cycle, the days leading up to ovulation. They stimulate the release of an egg from the ovary, which will then travel along the fallopian tube to the uterus. The point at which the egg leaves the ovary is ovulation and this occurs around fourteen days after the start of the last period. Some women are aware of having ovulated. They notice a slight change in their energy, or experience physical sensations. This can also be painful or cause discomfort, although most women do not notice anything.

After ovulation it is about fourteen days before bleeding starts. Each period is an opportunity for us to be reminded of our deep connection with other women, and with the natural world. A physical timeclock that marks the passage of our fertile days, always bringing us back to the possibility of exploring our own inner knowing. Today, however, it seems as though often the best that can be said about this potentially momentous occasion in every woman's life is if it can pass unnoticed. We seem to have lost touch with the magic of it, and be caught up in trying to make it all just disappear, like any other inconvenience.

The single most important thing that influences our experience of menstruation is attitude. In societies where it is honoured as a sacred time, one when a woman is in direct touch with the mysteries of life, period 'problems' tend to be minimal. In the absence of disease, our attitudes and our mother's attitudes towards bleeding can make every month a joyful celebration or an offensive intrusion.

Most women will notice a change in their energy shortly before a period is due. Feelings come closer to the surface, sensitivity is increased, along with intolerance, and awareness turns somehow inward. If we endeavour to suppress or ignore this change and carry on as usual, we can experience problems. Better to recognise and honour our changing focus, and show respect for our inner needs.

Managing Change

The moon is a marvellous symbol for the rhythms and changes of our own cycles. Every month it grows until it shines strong, clear and unmistakable in the night sky, then wanes until it is totally withdrawn, resting still and invisible before reappearing renewed and ready to commence the cycle again.

Many women find their menstrual flow appears either with the new moon or with the full moon. Traditionally, when a woman is ready to conceive, she will allow the light of the full moon to guide her to her lover, and bleed with the new moon. Similarly, when concentrating on inner work or other creative pursuits, she will tend to bleed with the new moon, using the strength of the full moon to fuel her creativity in other directions. This connection with the lunar cycle will also be influenced by the seasons, emotional factors and general health.

The moon controls tidal movement all over this planet, and has a direct effect on our body. Throughout many mysterious traditions, religions and faiths it has been connected with Women's Ways. The connection with the menstrual cycle is obvious, but it has also represented the quieter, more receptive, softer side of life, and been used as a symbol for feminine qualities and for the magical work that is best performed during the peace of the night.

Whenever a period comes, it is a good idea to reflect upon moon energy and the concept of the cycle, and use the event to gain insights into the current situation.

Take some time to yourself each month to connect with this experience and what it means for you. On a physical level your period may be just another biological event, yet emotionally and spiritually it can be much, much more than that.

Make a point, with each period, of spending some time in contact with nature. Be reminded of your connections to the elements and cycles of the world. Walk barefoot on a patch of clean grass or sand, and feel your connection with this Earth.

The time around each period is often when we become more aware of our own multi-faceted nature. Feelings and senses can become more acute and 'real' than usual as sensitivity increases. Our intuition and our emotions become more intense and unmistakable. This powerful time can make us feel much too vulnerable in a society where none of these factors are acknowledged, or are undervalued and unprotected. To Retreat at this time and honour our personal values is also to safeguard our ongoing health.

Planning a Retreat

This is an excellent way to honour yourself, your connectedness to other women and the natural world, and to explore fully the potential magic of your own experience of menstruation. Take some time off from your regular routine, and schedule time for your own needs, whatever you perceive them to be. It may be that it is time to bring more peace and stillness into your life, so relaxation, serenity and meditation would form the basis of your Retreat. Perhaps you need to allow your creativity and expressiveness, or your freedom of movement, or just need to be able to be, without having to do anything.

The Retreat can last for anything from one day, to as long as you can practically manage, or feel that you need. Many women find that three days is a good length, and enables them to replenish their energies and achieve their aims. The Retreat can offer a window into the stillness that is always at the centre of menstruation. Accessing this and the magic and mystery of this precious time can anchor us through seasons of emotional turmoil.

It is not often easy to justify that much time 'off' from a modern schedule, and it takes a real commitment to wanting to make this gift to yourself, to manage all the necessary arrangements. Work, and family, and other commitments of the ordinary world take precedence all month, and the point is that *sometimes you need to place your own needs foremost.*

Once you have made this commitment, it may well be that subsequent months will see you taking a much shorter, more manageable time out, and that symbols of your Retreat can be incorporated into your everyday life in the ordinary world that will support and further this inner process.

The real purpose of the Retreat is to put you back in touch with your own inner truths, so you need to exclude as many reminders of external reality as possible. It is a good idea to make this a solitary event, so exclude people by being alone, taking the telephone off the hook, and not going to places where you will be recognised and need to talk.

Avoid reading newspapers, books and magazines, and do not listen to the radio, television, or vocal music. Other reminders of time and commitments such as diaries, calendars and clocks may also be consigned to another place for the length of your Retreat.

Bring all that is positive and beautiful into your Retreat;

paintings, time in Nature, whatever you feel will enrich your experience. Plan to follow your own instinctive desires. Keep food simple, remember to drink lots, and let your own inner world be your guide – nap when you feel like, go outdoors when you feel like – release, and then allow yourself to be motivated by your own needs and sense of timing.

You will discover a wonderful sense of freedom as you begin to realise your own unbounded self. When your Retreat is over, prepare to enter the world again with increased creativity and inner calm, knowing you have been renewed and revitalised in some deep and uniquely personal way.

Your first Retreat is a wonderfully special occasion, akin to your first period. After it you are changed in some very real way. A fundamental shift will occur in your life when you begin to honour the flow of blood as a blessing.

You may also consider joining a group with other women who come together and share aspects of their experience, stories, and support. Recognising the commonality of all that we share can afford us a greater peace within ourselves as well as easier relationships with others. Moon groups such as these are a wonderful way to support your own individual growth.

Your Body Now

Take time to befriend your abdomen. Often when periods are an issue of discomfort our response is to shy away from that area of our body, whereas in fact the opposite can be most useful. Getting to know this part of your body will help you get in touch with your feminine side, and allay any fears or mystery surrounding your own experience of menstruation.

THE PELVIC BREATH

Choose a peaceful setting where you can be relaxed and undisturbed. Sit comfortably with your hands resting on your abdomen, and close your eyes. Take easy, gentle breaths right down into your pelvis, feeling the fresh air reach right down into your womb. Picture each breath as it extends down to the centre of your pelvis, bring light and energy with it, inspiring your whole body as it does so. Then picture any darkness, congestion, disharmony or tension leaving your body, on the breath, every time you breathe out. See the whole area around your womb clear, lighten, and be relieved of any pressures as you breathe gently and surely, relaxing deeply into the safety and security of your own energy.

Take your time and keep breathing in this way for as long as feels comfortable. Finish by taking a few large, deep breaths in, and stretching your body as you wake it up and breathe out. Consider spending fifteen or twenty minutes each day on this exercise.

THE PELVIC CIRCLE

This is a lovely thing to do on its own, or it can follow the Pelvic Breath (above). You will need some massage oil, and any type will do, or use olive, sesame or almond oil from the kitchen. If you like you can add two drops of any essential oil that appeals. Howood is a wonderfully scented pelvic decongestant, Rose is a strong uterine tonic and an utterly feminine scent, and Sandalwood is lovely for older skins, will support the kidneys and relieve any tensions.

Place the oil in a saucer or small bowl and warm gently by standing over a radiator or boiled saucepan of water for a few minutes.

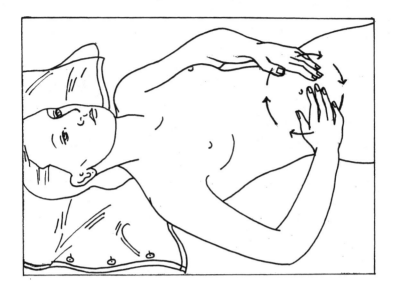

You can undress completely and uncover your pelvis, or just undress from the waist down. Lie down and get comfortable and place a pillow or cushion under your knees to relax your lower back. Place the oil beside you. Rest your hands palm down on your belly button. Close your eyes, and breathe easily deep down into your belly. Feel your relaxed hands gently rise and fall with each breath, and picture any surface tension or muscle-guarding melt away under the warm weight of your hands.

Take your time, and when you feel quite relaxed, remove one hand and soak it in the oil. Bringing it back to your belly button, start to make slow, gentle circles in a clockwise direction. Keep your eyes closed and feel your way. Involve your other hand, making slightly larger, soft circles around your belly button. With your hands working sometimes together, sometimes alternating, slowly extend the light circular touch until you are covering your whole pelvis.

Find for yourself what feels good, varying the speed to experience the touch differently. You may choose to linger in some spots, or enjoy the fluid feel of the overall rhythm. Keep the movements slow and gentle, and allow your hands to do whatever feels good, dipping them back into the oil whenever necessary. Let your hands stay relaxed, and keep your mind clear, allowing any images or pictures to enter and inform you.

You can do this for as long as feels comfortable, just remember to keep the rest of your body warm and relaxed. Finish by letting your hands rest on your belly button, and take a few more deep, cleansing breaths. Cover yourself and stay warm.

What to Eat Now

Food is an important area for women. We are traditionally the nurturers within our society, yet we receive some very mixed messages about how we are able to nourish and care for ourselves.

It is expected that we will take responsibility for the whole area of food preparation and presentation, but at the same time are made to feel we must be careful to limit and control the amount of food – which is, after all, positive nourishment – that we give to ourselves. The diet culture in which we live maintains that a 'good' food is one with little or no calorific content – one that has no energetic value. This means that the best food to give ourselves is one that has no value. So, what do we do when we have female children? This is such a strong wedge to place between women and their own power – their sense of connection with the earth, and their own position as nurturers – one could almost consider a conspiracy!

The entire subject can be pretty loaded, and it is important for our own health and well-being that we separate out the myth from the reality, and discover our own unique dietary requirements. There are all sorts of good health rules about eating some foods at different times, or combining certain foods; how regular mealtimes are essential, or how 'grazing' your way through the day is the best plan. They are all good guides if you use them to help you back to your own needs. In a culture that grows on uniformity, it is a well-kept secret that all our needs are slightly different. And what nobody ever told you (unless you were very lucky) is that it is your job to discover what works best for you.

Keeping a diet diary is a good way to begin to tease out our own physical and emotional responses to food.

KEEPING A DIET DIARY

This is a wonderful way to really get to know our eating habits, and to explore some of the connections between what we eat and how we feel. The best way to do this is to record absolutely everything that is eaten and drunk every day for at least one week, ideally for a month. Make a daily sheet for yourself, and note down:

- What you eat and drink
- The time and place
- Whether alone or in company
- How you feel
- Physical symptoms

Repeat this for every meal or snack and then collate the information, reviewing it daily and at the end of the week.

How you feel when you are eating will govern how well your food is absorbed and just how much nourishment you are getting from each meal. The stark truth is that within the bounds of a healthy basic diet, if you feel relaxed and happy and take each meal in good company, then you are least likely to experience any food-related intolerance, allergy or other symptoms. Keeping your own diet diary will let you see clearly how close you come to that ideal, and should also help pin-point your own emotional patterns around eating and nourishing yourself. It will also shed light on how well you mix food groups and how balanced your diet is.

Both appetite and dietary needs change throughout the monthly cycle. Just before each period, our calorie needs may increase by up to 500 calories (2.09kJ) a day. This can represent an increase of up to 50 per cent of some women's everyday intake. It is important to recognise our own changing needs, and respect the body's signs and signals.

The first time I saw Melanie, a twenty-five-year-old professional, she could hardly sit up straight from the pain of menstrual cramps. She looked pale and wan, with big dark circles under her eyes, and seemed to have no energy at all. Her period had just begun, and already that day she had skipped breakfast, but eaten three bars of chocolate, wanting the energy without the feeling of fullness in her stomach.

I sent her home to get into bed with a hot water bottle and some warming soup, to ride out the pains, and get as much rest as she could. As soon as she was able to get around, we launched into a month of strengthening and warming activity to influence the next period. She started to eat a large, warming breakfast every day, although at first it was all she could manage to pick at some soup or a boiled egg. Lunch was also a cooked meal, with a warming soup for supper. She took a multivitamin and mineral supplement every day, and also had a cup of yarrow tea. She was under strict instructions to keep her feet warm, and avoid draughts – her tendency had always been to walk around barefoot, even in the coldest winter months.

After two weeks of this, she was still struggling with eating warm foods early in the day, and felt rather stifled by keeping wrapped up with clothes all the time. We persevered, and I suggested a vigorous exercise routine as another way of keeping warm. She began slowly, but by the time her period was due, managed to do ten minutes every day of some sort of exercise. Her sugar cravings were noticeably different, she found that she only wanted something really sweet if she was late having a meal. The day her period began was the only time she had chocolate that month.

Her next period was considerably less painful, and she managed to go to work every day, rather than needing at least two days off. By the beginning of her next cycle she was waking up hungry for food, and was able to include all the additional foods I had suggested to warm her up and treat her spleen (yellow foods like squash, sweet potato, corn and carrots). She was generally feeling stronger, and her weak kidneys were responding to the yarrow tea – she no longer paid lots of visits to the loo each day and night. She was enjoying the exercise, and looked altogether like a different woman. Her next period was considerably better again, with minimal cramps, and the sugar cravings had all but disappeared.

Food cravings are one of the ways that the body can use to draw our attention to specific shortfalls in the diet. Trusting your body in this way requires you to fly in the face of conventional thinking, and invest in the belief that your body is your friend and wants only the best for you. The pay-off can be wonderful in terms of renewed health and vitality, and an increasing feeling of physical safety and security as you discover the powerful ally that you have in yourself.

Many of us experience dietary cravings before each period, and these can provide strong clues to our overall nutritional deficiencies, as well as to any immediate health needs. Sugar cravings occur when our energy needs peak in our physical efforts to make the period happen (see p.95). If any of these appear familiar, consult a practitioner for individual advice, or consider supplementing the diet with rich sources of the specific nutrient for a month or two, and seeing whether any changes occur.

A craving for bananas could point to an overall potassium deficiency. Good dietary sources include parsley, horseradish, cress and sweet potatoes. Craving cheese could pin-point calcium needs, so add extra sesame seeds, almonds and rosehips to the diet throughout the month. Chocolate cravings can be the result of a magnesium deficiency, so increase dietary broccoli, chickpeas, chives and fennel leaves. If you get cravings for green vegetables, eat more – this can be because of a phosphorus, iodine or chlorophyll deficiency. Other good food sources include sea vegetables and seaweeds.

Staying Well

*   Regular Sitz Baths are a wonderful, invigorating way to ensure good tone throughout the entire pelvic region. Take once a month, or more in response to any specific complaints.

SITZ BATHS

Method 1 (with a portable shower head)

Fill the bath to mid-calf level with cold water. Step in, and turn on the shower head with the water running very warm. Shower all around your pelvis, across the hips, over your bottom and in between the legs for about two minutes. Turn off the shower and sit down in the bath, so that both your feet and your bottom are immersed in the cool water. After one minute, stand up carefully and run the shower with very warm water, again covering the pelvis region as before and making sure to pass it all around the hips and through the legs. Spray for about one minute then turn off the water and sit down once more in the bath.

After about two minutes, pull out the plug and let the water drain away. Stand up carefully just as soon as you are ready and wrap yourself in a warm towel. Rest for at least five minutes and then take a warm drink.

Method 2 (if you do not have a shower spray)

This follows the same plan as method 1, only a container such as a baby bath or a large washing-up bowl is used in place of the shower spray.

Fill the bath, as before, to about mid-calf level with cold water. Place the container containing hot water into the bath. Repeat the process as above, this time adjusting your sitting position so that you spend two minutes in the hot water with your feet in cold. Then switch to sit in the cold water of the bath, with your feet in the container of hot water for about one minute. Repeat the move, and then finish by sitting down in the cold water for about one minute.

Sit out on the side of the bath wrapped in a towel for a few minutes, then rest for at least five minutes before having a warm drink.

• Internal sanitary protection is a choice for many women,

although this can irritate and prolong the flow of bleeding. The presence of a strange body of matter in the vagina may also create changes in the local acidity and allow a route for infection, or allow inflammation to occur. External protection is a more positive choice, and is recommended whenever there are menstrual difficulties. It is also important to ensure its use overnight whilst sleeping.

Small pieces of natural sponge make a handy alternative to tampons when internal protection is essential. Dampen before use to avoid scratching the vaginal walls, and simply rinse well in hot water and reinsert as needed. These small sponges are often sold as beauty accessories, and are good for applying foundation. You can sew in a short length of thread if you are concerned about removal, although if you keep the sponge close to the vaginal entry this should not really be necessary. Make sure you change or rinse the sponge regularly throughout the day.

Managing stress

Spend some time today thinking about the types of situation in which you feel pressured or stressed. Consider the things that have troubled you and occasions on which you actually noticed being tense.

Make a list of six times that you think of recently when you have been stressed or uncomfortable. Try to recall how you felt physically – were there any places in particular that you noticed become tight, or sore, or any overall feelings such as a headache, or a sensation like energy, or exhilaration, or fear. Re-run the events in your mind and recall how they made you feel. Note, too, how they affected you emotionally – did you notice any feelings? See if you can remember how long they lasted, and whether your mind remained clear, and any other things that are part of the way you respond to stress.

Now assess what might have helped you feel better – carry on running the image in your mind, and see for yourself which strategies work best. Consider taking a deep breath, dropping your shoulders, unclenching your jaw or fist, or simply moving into another position. Wriggling your toes can help because it focuses your body's attention and draws energy down from the biggest potential trouble spots of the face, neck and shoulders. Shifting tension often requires only a small move, and consciously relaxing can be enough to change the whole pattern of stress in your body.

It is important to know what techniques work for you. Replaying the range of potential solutions to stressful scenarios, in your mind's eye, lets you find out. It can also prepare you for the next time you face a similar situation, and equips you with an armoury of stress-busters so that you always have a mechanism up your sleeve to cope with any difficult situation.

Finish this exercise by listing six things that you find really relaxing and enjoyable – anything at all, from spending time alone, to dancing, listening to birds in the morning, taking a bath by candlelight, receiving a relaxing massage, or taking a stroll at twilight. List whatever relaxes you, and then take your diary and schedule in some time over the next two weeks to spend time doing just those things.

TONING

This is an exercise aimed specifically at expelling disharmony from the body and changing energy in a surprisingly effective way. Do this every day:

- to harmonise the body;

- to free up this style of expressing yourself;
- as part of a meditation practice;
- or for the simple pleasure it brings.

Start by sitting comfortably and taking a few deep, relaxing breaths. Choose a vowel sound (a, ay, ee, o, oo, etc.) and any note you like. Breathe deep down into your body and, as you exhale, let the air come out with the sound you have chosen. Do not force your breath or look for projection, or any great resonance, or even to hold pitch, simply let out the sound. Keeping your breathing continuous make your sound with each exhalation.

You will find that the note you are singing and the sound you make, will change as you continue the exercise. Follow your body's lead and allow the sound to modulate as it needs to. Just open your mouth and allow a noise to come out. You will find that the sound eventually sweetens or becomes more harmonious, so by the end of the exercise you will be making and hearing the healing tones that your body needs to rebalance itself.

You can strengthen the effect of the exercise by covering the energy centre just below your belly button with your left hand, and resting your right hand loosely over it. This centre of physical energy and balance is sited a few fingers width below your belly button, and covering it with relaxed hands will focus your breathing.

If you are feeling 'under the weather' or have a specific health complaint, Toning is a powerful way to change the energy and address any dysfunction. I find this especially useful for warding off colds and tiredness, and also for shifting blockages in the body such as in constipation, late menstruation, and dry coughs, as well as when there is an inability to express yourself in some way.

To Tone to address specific difficulties, begin as before by relaxing then close your eyes and see your breath entering the part of the body in difficulty. Make sure that each breath you take reaches right into the centre of this place, then breathe out from there making any sound that your body needs to – maybe a vowel sound, or a sigh, a whine or a groan. Keep your breathing continuous and observe how the sound changes, until you reach a natural close.

You can also use this as a dynamic technique to move emotional or creative blocks, by breathing into different areas of your emotional world, or Toning while replaying scenes in your mind. Always finish by taking a couple of full, deep breaths, and consciously relaxing all over as you breathe out any residual tension or tiredness. Shrug your shoulders a few times and wriggle your toes. Take another deep breath and as you breathe out gently stretch out your arms and legs, then sit quietly for a moment.

Sugar cravings

These commonly occur before a period, and are almost always a symptom of nutritional deficiency. If left unchecked, they can become a problem throughout the month. The body's response to sugar is instant. It tastes great, and gives you an immediate energy lift. It could easily be regarded as a powerful stimulant drug because of its strong and addictive effect. In common with tea, caffeine and alcohol, the other stimulants regularly found in our diet, we quite soon feel the need for more and more frequent doses.

Every time your body's sugar levels rise to a peak in response to the sugar you eat, there is a subsequent drop in energy levels that follows as surely as night follows day. It is very easy to respond to this energy slump by taking more sugar, and that is the worst possible habit to set up.

Breaking the pattern requires some application but is well worth it, both in terms of the physical relief it brings, and the satisfaction of knowing that you have faced an addiction. Follow the guidelines below, and consider consulting your practitioner to work more with your own individual nutritional status.

- Plan regular mealtimes and stick to them. This ensures a regular supply of energy for your body.
- Plan at least five small meals each day instead of the usual two or three large ones. This will maintain your blood sugar levels.
- Avoid stimulants that will upset your body's balance even further, e.g. alcohol, cigarettes, coffee, cola and tea.
- Increase the amount of fresh fruit and vegetables that you eat. This will provide your body with more energy as well as valuable nutrients.
- Exercise and spend some time outdoors every day.
- Keep a supply of protein-based snacks to hand for the first month. Take whenever sugar cravings appear, or energy levels drop. Consider nuts, seeds (sunflower are especially good), cooked chicken or shellfish, cheese, burgers, e.g. soya and lentil, beansprouts, etc.
- In the week before your period is due, amend your diet still further so that you have some carbohydrate, even if it is just a slice of toast, a biscuit, banana or crispbread, every two hours.

Absent periods

Any absence of periods should always be checked out. Leaving aside the possibility of pregnancy, this could point to the possibility of an hormonal imbalance that will respond well if treated early. An absence of periods in the 30s may indicate the beginning of an irregular pattern, that will lead to the menopause. Once past 35, it is not uncommon to skip an occasional period, and this is especially the case during times of emotional upset or upheaval.

If you can pin-point an ovulation time, then treat immediately by following a mono-diet or fruit fast for three days. This means you choose a type of fruit and eat only large amounts of this, and drink lots and lots of water for those three days. If no ovulation is found, follow the moon. You can assume ovulation is occurring with the new moon, and follow the food plan then. Take a Sitz Bath every other day until the full moon (when bleeding could be expected), and practise some form of Retreat at that time. Monitor your appetite for any cravings that may point towards dietary imbalance, and consider taking an all-round vitamin and mineral supplement. If you do not respond to this after three months, seek the advice of your practitioner or healer.

PMS – Pre-menstrual syndrome

This is also known as PMT or pre-menstrual tension. It is called a syndrome because it embraces a wide range of symptoms. These are hormonal in origin, and almost always disappear once the period starts. Nutrition pays an important note here. Some women experience this syndrome every month, and others on occasion. The symptoms vary in intensity, and some months may be better than others. The symptoms can be both physical and emotional, and include water retention with breast tenderness and abdominal distension, headaches, fainting, irritability, depression and mood swings. Tiredness, sugar cravings, nervous tension and back pain complete the picture, although there are other difficulties that can also fit.

The best treatment is to get the whole body back to total health, while treating the worst of the symptoms. Follow a good basic diet to redress any nutritional imbalances, and ensure you eat plenty of fresh fruit and vegetables, preferably organically grown, and cut out all stimulants including tea, salt, sugar and chocolate. This will let your system begin to rebalance itself. Do not smoke, and be careful to reduce the amount of pollution you expose yourself to. Consider a supplement of pycnogenol and some stress-buster B-vitamins to counteract the effects of living with excess stress. Learn to relax in whatever way works best for you.

If symptoms persist or there is no improvement, consult your healthcare practitioner.

Fluid retention

The discomfort of bloating and water retention will recede if you increase the amount of water that you drink each day, and reduce all foods that will hold water in the body. Avoid meats and salty tastes, increasing the amount of lightly cooked vegetables that you eat and include some natural diuretics like parsley, cooked fennel bulb and celery. Gently warm the body by adding cinnamon, turmeric and small amounts of ginger to meals, and drink warm herbal teas throughout the day.

Headaches

Tension headaches may well respond to relaxation techniques or to the occasional massage to relieve the neck and shoulder area. Once the bowel is clear, congestive headaches tend to disappear, so treat by drinking lots of water, and eating stewed mung beans, seasoned with ginger, cinnamon and garlic, with rice every day. If the discomfort is severe, make a paste from water and a little ginger powder, and place on the piece of bone at the bottom of the ear just under the lobe. You can repeat this up to three times in any one day, but once will usually be enough.

Fainting

This is not a normal occurrence. If it occurs regularly at the onset, or just before the period is due, then consult your practitioner. Often when the hormonal balance is in difficulty, the additional energy it takes to begin the period can create an enormous amount of internal heat leading to sweats and fainting.

Efforts to cool the body in the fortnight leading up to the period will prove fruitful. Avoid eating meat, spicy foods like chilli, and foods that are very sour like vinegar and tomatoes. Do not drink alcohol or coffee, and reduce carbonated drinks. Keep some cool peppermint, fennel or liquorice root tea on hand and drink at least three cups each day. See also Heavy Periods (p.104) because anaemia can cause fainting.

If feelings of weakness and fragility occur throughout the month, a constitutional treatment needs to be sought. In this case take care to strengthen and warm the body by eating warm, cooked foods and drinks, keeping the body warm, particularly around the pelvis, and adding small amounts of warming spices to the diet, like cinnamon and clove.

Irritability, depression and mood swings

Meditate or find some time for quiet contemplation each morning. Make it your focus to remember that you can retain your equilibrium, whatever the circumstances, and that there is always a still centre at the very core of your being. Chew a handful of fennel seeds, and take cool fennel or liquorice root tea if you find yourself becoming emotionally heated. Introduce some time each day when you can walk barefoot on a patch of clean grass and renew your inner coolness, and your connection with the rest of the natural world. Consult your practitioner for further personalised advice, and use affirmations to achieve the change you need.

Back pain

This is common just before bleeding starts, or for the first day or so of the period. Eating stewed mung beans seasoned with garlic, ginger and cinnamon, and rice as the main meal once a day for the week when the period is due will help. This will remove any bowel obstruction and soften the lower back. Make sure you drink lots of water too, to ensure soft and regular bowel movements.

Make sure that posture is good, and that there is not a structural problem – consider having an osteopathic check-up. Methods for reducing water retention will help relieve any pressure on the lower back, and the Pelvic Tilt position (see p.103) should offer immediate relief.

Tiredness

Having a period is quite a tiring thing for the body to do, particularly as it gets older. Often an extra hour's sleep at night, or a short nap in the day will be enough to see off any tiredness. If it is severe, check overall nutrition, and ensure that the period is not too heavy. Low iron levels resulting from heavy blood loss can lead to tiredness (see p.104). Ensure a regular intake of small carbohydrate meals every day in the week leading up to menstruation, and take 1g (1,000mg) of vitamin C each day of the cycle leading up to the next period. Take the tissue salt combination B for an immediate answer to tiredness.

Painful periods

Many women experience a small amount of cramping just as each period begins. It this is severe, prolonged, or begins after the period has started, it is recommended that you consult your healthcare practitioner. Pain like this is not an inevitable part of menstruation, and there is much that can be done to redress any individual imbalance.

In the meantime, keep your pelvis warm (make a sandwich of it between two hot water bottles) and have plenty of fresh air. Take a tea made from two parts Lady's mantle and one part yarrow, by steeping a teaspoonful in boiling water for about thirty seconds. Sip this slowly while it is still hot and take twice a day until the pain lifts or you contact your practitioner. This may also be taken once a day for the three days around ovulation, and for the three days before the next period is due as a preventative measure. Consider the tissue salt Mag. Phos., or Combination N, as emergency first aid.

Make sure the bowel is clear. Often constipation will add to feelings of congestion and can cause pain itself. One of the best ways to ensure regular bowel movements is to eat stewed mung beans seasoned with garlic, ginger, and cinnamon, with rice for two or three days when the period is due. If this is not possible, increase the amount of fresh fruit and vegetables you eat, and keep food warm, avoiding anything that is chilled or frozen like ice-cream. Eat mainly cooked meals, drink hot water with each meal, or add warming spices such as ginger and cinnamon. It is also important to drink large amounts of water. This will help keep the bowels clear, and will also relieve any mild nausea. For an immediate laxative, take one teaspoon of ghee in a glass of warm milk before bedtime, and it will work first thing in the morning. (Do not repeat this more than once a month.)

Katy, a strong, energetic forty-five-year-old was in good general health, but plagued by period cramps that lasted for the first two days of her flow every month, and were violent enough to incapacitate her. She bled very heavily during those first two days, and then settled down to a normal flow.

She had been using Clary Sage essential oil to massage her abdomen as soon as the cramping began, and this was encouraging the heavy flow. I recommended that she take the tissue salt Mag. Phos. every day throughout the first month, increasing the dose when her period came due. The Clary Sage oil was to be used in a simple compress (made by soaking a strip of clean cotton fabric in a bowl of hot water to which two drops of the essential oil had been added). I suggested she place this over her pelvis and replace it as soon as it cooled, but only once the cramping had begun, and just before bedtime each evening.

Her first period showed no change, but Katy persevered and by the third month was experiencing an improvement of about 80 per cent. She continued to take the tissue salt with each period, only when cramping began, and it worked very quickly to bring relief.

The Pelvic Circle exercise (see p.84) is a very good idea. Make some time to do this when your period is due, perhaps the evening before it starts. If it has already arrived and is sore, add two drops of Dr Bach's Crab Apple or Rescue Remedy to the oil, and make sure the oil is nice and warm before you begin. You may also like to wrap a hot water bottle in a towel and keep it next to you, or lie with your bottom on it while you massage your abdomen.

PELVIC TILT

This is an excellent position for instant pain relief. You can do this almost anywhere and the positive effects do last for a short time after you get up.

Kneel down on the floor or on the bed, and place your hands down flat in front of you. Keep your legs from your knees to your ankles parallel, and a few inches apart. Bend your arms and slowly lower your upper body until your chest is flat on the floor (or bed). Turn your head to one side to make breathing easier, and remain in this position for as long as you like. It is surprisingly comfortable, and brings relief quite speedily.

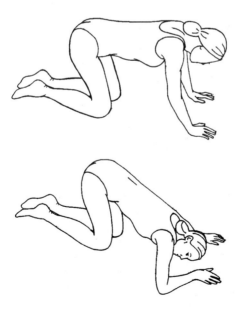

Heavy periods

Heavy or prolonged blood loss can be a tremendous drain, leaving you feeling exhausted and sickly after every period. The heavy flow can also be difficult to manage on a practical level, leaving some women almost housebound every month.

Anaemia can become a problem if bleeding is excessive or when heavy periods are a regular occurrence, and iron stores are depleted. Symptoms include headaches, tiredness, lethargy and pallor. You may also notice nails becoming brittle and a sore mouth and tongue. A blood test will confirm any suspicions.

Stop wearing internal protection straight away. Take silica (as a supplement) and make sure the diet contains many iron-rich foods. These include organically reared animal flesh, egg yolk, peas, beans and lentils, molasses, shellfish, parsley, nuts, watercress, green leafy vegetables, dandelion leaves, nettles, elderberries, sorrel and coriander leaves or cilantro. Vitamins C and E enhance iron absorption. Drink one large glass of beetroot juice each day, and add raw beetroot to your diet.

Resources
The Wise Wound Penelope Shuttle and Peter Redgrove, Paladin
The 13 Original Clan Mothers Jamie Sams, HarperCollins
Beat PMS Through Diet Dr Michelle Harrison, Optima
Moon Time Johanna Paungger and Thomas Poppe, C. W. Daniel

PMS Help PO Box 160, St Albans, AL1 4YQ

Women's Nutritional Advisory Service PO Box 268, Lewes, East Sussex BN7 2QN. 01273 487366

SEXUAL MATURITY

Once through puberty, the sexual characteristics of growing breasts, pubic hair, changing body shape and menstruation appear. This means we are reaching sexual maturity. Our bodies reach a time of sexual ability, however, often long before we have the emotional maturity to embrace our sexuality and make informed choices about it. Whatever our decisions about sexual activity, this is a time to take responsibility for ourselves, to look after our bodies and instigate regular health checks. It is the beginning of our exploration of the complex world of relationships, and the dawn of our expression of love and tenderness in a new experience of intimacy.

The strength and intensity of sexual passion can be overwhelming or a little frightening at times. This is surely one of the reasons that so much emphasis is placed on sexual behaviour by different religions and societies. Fear is at the root of many of the restrictions that prevent women from expressing their sexuality. It is also the basis for many of the prejudices that exist towards those who embrace and express their sexuality, or who do so in seemingly unconventional ways. Cultural expectation and religious and family teachings inform our attitudes long before we are in a position to experience our own choices. Sexual energy is a vital part of our lives, and the continued life of our species depends upon it. We are all sexual beings, and we have a choice about whether and how to express that energy.

For some women, sexuality is a quiet, wholly intimate matter, and for others a more social affair to be openly explored and experimented with. Our health depends upon us being easy and comfortable with this as with every other aspect of our nature. To be sexually aware is to understand our own body energy, whether or not to be sexually active is an individual choice.

Sexuality touches upon many other needs and areas of our lives. We all have a need for intimacy, and our skins can thirst for touch. The erotic in our lives and our sensual nature also longs to be explored. This makes for a pretty heady mix. Deciding which elements can or need to be separated or explored can be quite a task. Love and sex are a traditional pairing, so are sex and power, and love and marriage. It can seem as though to separate love and sex would diminish both, yet there are extremely successful celibate relationships, and some marriages embrace a degree of sexual promiscuity. It seems it is certainly possible to separate physical expression from our emotions and feelings; we must decide for ourselves whether or not this is desirable.

Today many people question whether it is good to be sexually active. Some feel that the power of sexuality needs to be contained within the bounds of a committed relationship. It is important to women's health that we are free to make our own choices.

Managing Change

We need to know our own sexual limits or boundaries in order to feel comfortable within ourselves. By being honest with ourselves about our needs and desires, we can begin to enter into relationship with others. Considering whether, when and with whom to have sex is a very big question. Celibacy is a choice for an increasing number of women today, both in and out of relationships. There is also an increasing trend for girls to maintain their virginity before settling down with a life partner, although this is often as a reaction to the increasing severity of sexually transmitted diseases. Serial monogamy seems to be a very common choice too, although this can feel like a compromise; on the other hand, there is an increasing number of purely sexual relationships. In fact, there is a multiplicity of patterns of relationship, and what is important is finding what works best for you: it seems that there has rarely been more freedom to pursue whatever type of sexual expression best suits you.

Sexual appetites differ between individuals, and will alter through each menstrual cycle and at different times in our lives. Our expression and orientation are as uniquely individual as any other of our character traits. Whether we feel free to experiment with sexual freedom or need to feel certain constraints in order to liberate our appetite and passion, intimacy is always possible.

Whenever we come close to another individual in this way, we open lots of doors for ourselves. Becoming so exquisitely vulnerable with another person, finding that degree of trust, reaching such passionate heights and finally letting go in the release of a climax are all pretty amazing things for us to do. Lovers are usually the only people who see us naked. We are all aware of how beautiful bodies can be, and yet it is common for us as women to feel that our own bodies are less than adequate in some way, or to be overly aware of what we perceive to be our own imperfections. To bare all, then, to another, is a wonderfully generous action. It is to tell a huge secret, to take a big risk, and actually it is to show and share our own divinity.

The last people who were close too you when you were naked and vulnerable were your parents or carers. Often close relationships can remind us of any unfinished emotional business that we are carrying from our childhood, or from earlier relationships. This sort of emotional baggage can colour our physical responses, and influence relationships. It is worth reviewing your own personal history to see whether you are carrying anything else with you when you are with your lover, or whether indeed anyone else is there too.

These days there are other implications of sexual intimacy that we need to consider. Alongside the potential for unplanned pregnancy, unprotected sex can have serious health risks. More and more couples are choosing to enjoy safer sex, even within established relationships, and this not only protects as much as possible against the HIV and other viruses, but also increases communication between lovers. It also opens the doors to a different type of sexual activity, one that is less motivated by penetration or intercourse, and that can concentrate on giving and receiving other sexual pleasures. Intimacy is not reliant upon sexual intercourse, and this is the most important or satisfying aspect of sexual relations. The intimacy of a close relationship is many times better than unsatisfactory sex.

Orgasms appear to be a matter of great contention. Some women have difficulty experiencing orgasm at all, others worry that they do not experience multiple orgasms, or that they take too long to climax, or that they orgasm too soon. Learning to relax and trust the body, and the situation that we are in, makes it easier to accept our own sexual style and response. Some people are quick to anger, burst into explosive laughter, and have strong physical reactions, while others are slower to respond, taking time to get the joke or to be stirred into action; so it is with our sexuality.

It serves little purpose to compare sexual reaction times or achievements. If you are happy with your orgasm then that is wonderful. If you do not experience a climax and are happy that too is just fine. If you want to experience a climax, or want one more quickly or more slowly, then you can experiment with any number of enjoyable ways of changing your sexual practices.

Fantasy is an important element for many women. It is often a key to experiencing orgasm when alone, and may figure in shared sexual activity in a private way or as part of a game that is played together. Sexual fantasising is just the same as day dreaming, only with a different subject matter. It can be about anything that you find appealing and stimulating, from kissing your partner to something much raunchier. Props such as appealing underwear and sexual toys can also be part of exploring orgasms. A number of women find that they get turned on by wearing or not wearing certain pieces of clothing.

Many aspects of our sexual nature can be experienced on our own, and some require us to be with a partner. If we do not know for ourselves what will bring us to orgasm it is difficult to expect anybody else to. Pleasuring ourselves is the beginning of understanding what we like and what we don't like, which makes it easier to communicate that comfortably to a lover. Masturbation is a perfectly normal part of life.

Relaxation is important to many orgasms. The more pressure you feel because this is something that you don't often do, or because you are unsure how, or uncertain about the situation you are in, the harder it is for your body to let go. Practise some good physical relaxation techniques that will enable you to feel comfortable with letting go to the good sensations in your body. The sexual breath is a powerful technique that can begin to open up this area of experience, and is worth persevering with. Do it regularly and to begin with only do it when you are on your own.

SEXUAL BREATH

Spend five to ten minutes each day relaxing and breathing deeply right into your vulva. Imagine each breath reaching right down into that place, and just be aware of the sensations it brings. Breathe out from there too, bringing the breath up right through the body and out, being aware of how connected your genitals are with the rest of your body. Get to know the feelings and sensations of being connected to your vulva.

Continue breathing deeply as your vaginal lips begin to soften and fill, and a general warmth suffuses the whole region. Allow the whole area between your legs to soften and glisten with sweet moisture as you relax and simply breathe into that part of your body.

Keep your breathing going and as rhythmic and fluid as possible. After about ten minutes, place both hands on your abdomen and take some easy, relaxed breaths as you return to your normal breathing pattern. Take a few moments to rest and review what has just occurred.

Many women find this becomes exciting, and can be a prelude to sex. This is a technique that can also be shared with your partner.

Often the first thing to go obviously 'wrong' in a relationship is the sex. If you are in a sexual relationship that is not working on any level, your body may well be the most obvious way to let you know. If your sexual response to a partner is unfailingly withdrawn, stilted or ceases to be pleasurable, then you may find that the root of the difficulty is in other areas of your relationship. If you can continue to find pleasure and reach a climax on your own but not with your partner, then maybe they do not know how to pleasure you. Communication is very important between lovers just as in any other type of relationship, and improving this aspect of the relationship can heighten all aspects of it.

Your Body Now

Sex involves the whole body. It is certainly not just centred in the genitals. You can experiment with this for yourself by noticing just how excited you can become while avoiding genital stimulation. Many women know that any kind of touch, even holding hands, or just standing and looking at someone, can be as much of a turn-on as anything else if the time is right, and the person is right. Expanding sexual awareness or activity to include the whole body acknowledges what we have always really known to be true and deeply enriches our sexual experience.

Experiment for yourself with using different types of touch either on your own or with your lover. Experience the all-over pleasure of being touched and stroked using just one finger, or a tongue. Close your eyes to intensify the physical sensation. Cover the body using a silk pad, or the light touch of a feather. Delicately stroke your body with a fresh flower or a sprig of fresh fragrant herbs such as lavender, rosemary or thyme.

As women we have a highly developed sensual side which deserves to be explored. This is what allows us to experience pleasure without necessarily crossing the border into sexuality. That boundary is often hard to define, and investigating it can be a wonderfully pleasurable pursuit.

In a society that both prices and fears women's sexuality, this type of physical pursuit has often been proscribed because of the danger it poses. As we regain sovereignty of our own bodies, knowledge of what pleases and pleasures us can be very empowering.

There are many simple ways in which nature can aid our exploration of this aspect of ourselves either on our own or with another. For sheer pleasure, find a safe place where you will be able to lie naked on a patch of grass for a short time. Close your eyes and feel the sun warm and slowly fill your skin, while the breeze gently touches your whole body, stimulating nerve endings and generating an incredible natural high. If you have ever been swimming without any clothes on, you will have been able to feel the all-over delight of the water touching and supporting all your body. It is well worth seeking out experiences like this to add to your life.

Massage is a wonderful way to pleasure the body. It can be an excellent remedial therapy for dealing with tension and structural difficulties, and may also be the medium for introducing aromatherapy and other remedies to the body. Specifically sensual massage is a delightful way for lovers to increase their communication and enjoy each other's bodies. You can massage yourself, visit a professional massage therapist, or have a partner do it for you. All will be very different experiences. Having a professional massage might give you some tips about different strokes and techniques that you can use yourself.

To massage yourself, simply find a comfortable position in which you can relax, and begin by gently stroking whatever body part you have chosen. You can just use the flat of your hands, or your fingers, and repeated, rhythmic strokes will be easy to do and feel good. Later you can expand and experiment with varying the pressure and speed of the strokes, and with using a light lifting motion, or using just your finger tips with a percussive movement that feels like raindrops falling on the skin. For now just allow your hands to relax and follow the contours of your body.

Legs and arms, the chest and abdomen, the face and head are all easy to reach, as are the hands and arms. Reaching the shoulders and parts of the back can be done with the aid of a few pillows to prop yourself up. This is a lovely way to deepen your own connection with your body, and feels quite different to when anybody else does it for you. If you do have somebody else massage you, you will be able to relax more, but in a different way. Experience this for yourself if you are able to enjoy both. Always remember to be as relaxed as possible, and not to use any pressure, particularly on the abdomen.

You can use oil or cream to massage with, and this will make it different yet again. Add essential oils to the mix for an aromatherapy massage that will enhance the experience and pleasure another sense. Sesame, almond, and rape seed oils are good for massage, but any oil can be used including olive and even vegetable oil from the kitchen.

Pour a small amount of the oil into a saucer or shallow dish, and place on a radiator or over a saucepan of warm water for a few moments so that it is not too cold. Never pour the oil onto your skin, always take it up onto your hands first, this makes sure the oil is at the right temperature, and makes it easier to work, and less messy.

Add two drops of an essential oil to make this a sensual aromatherapy massage. Choose any fragrance that you like, bearing in mind the attributes and associations of each oil. Ylang-ylang is a definite aphrodisiac, Rose enhances the feminine aspects, and Sandalwood aids relaxation as well as being very good for the skin.

Sally was an elegant-looking woman in her mid-30s, who neverthe-less appeared to be keeping her ears warm with her shoulders – they were held so high and tight. She took a long time to tell me about her area of difficulty, alluding to some sort of physical or sexual prob-lem without saying exactly what it was, and detailing some minor physical complaints to skirt away from the subject. When she finally managed to tell me that she could not reach orgasms with her part-ner, the sense of relief in the room was palpable.

She was rather shy about her body, and in fact found it difficult even to discuss other physical functions like menstruation. Her whole physical attitude was rather as though she was distancing herself as much as she possibly could from her pelvis, and I wondered how dif-ficult the whole sexual experience must be for her. She admitted that she found it all slightly distasteful, but felt that she needed to include it to be fully in the relationship.

We began by learning some exercises to encourage her to breathe fully into her body, and to begin to touch herself lovingly all over. Over the next two months we introduced physical exercises to increase her sense of being in her body, and she also found a local massage therapist and had a weekly massage. We strengthened her diet to include more roughage and natural fibre from fresh fruit and vegetables so that her pelvis would be clear and bowel movements easier.

The two most useful measures were in encouraging her to dis-cuss this freely with her boyfriend (she practised with me, then in front of a mirror, and finally talked about it with him) and suggesting that she obtain some literature or videos about sexual relationships to see whether she might not start to feel more relaxed about it all once she was more *au fait* with what was going on. She also learned some specific exercises to loosen up her lower back and breathe into her pelvis.

Six months after her consultation, Sally had her first orgasm with her boyfriend, and I understand that things have continued to improve.

Breast examination

It is important to do this regularly, every month. Choose a time a few days after your period has ended, because breasts will often feel a little enlarged and more tender before menstruation.

Begin by observing your breasts in a mirror. Look at the way they sit on your chest from the front and the side. Observe your nipples and the way they appear. Then lean forward from the waist and look at the way your breasts hang forward. You are getting to know what looks normal for you, and learning how smooth, symmetrical and full each breast is. Any changes in this appearance should prompt you to consult your practitioner.

Now lie down on your back with an extra small pillow under your left shoulder. Using the flat of your right hand, feel all around the area of your left breast, from the armpit to the middle of your sternum, and from just below your collar bone to the ribs below your breast. Now you are getting a feel for the whole region, and seeing how soft, mobile, and heavy the breast is.

Work your way all over your left breast, pressing down slightly to feel the muscular supports, and make small circular movements to check all round the area up to your nipple. Be gentle and take your time. It is absolutely fine to be excited or stimulated by this, but pay attention to the task.

Once you have covered the whole of your left breast and the surrounding area, change sides. Place the small pillow

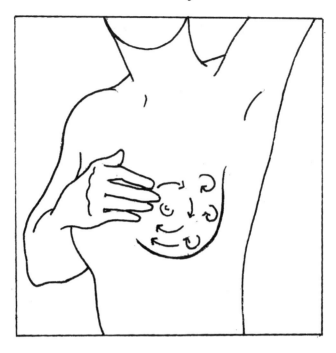

under your right shoulder, and using the flat of your left hand with a firm but gentle touch, repeat the process for your right breast.

For the first few months you will probably just be building a picture of what is normal for you. Then you will be able to spot any changes quickly. Look for anything that is out of the ordinary for you, including areas of tenderness, changes in appearance, and any alterations in texture. Some breasts are very glandular, and can feel a little 'lumpy' all the time. If you are in any doubt about what you are feeling, consult your practitioner. They will be able to check that you are doing this in the best possible way, and answer any questions that you may have, or examine your breasts for you.

Breast appearance, texture and fullness can all change in

response to a host of different things, including age and the season, body weight, where in the monthly cycle you are, and whether you have a lover. (A surprising number of breast lumps are first discovered by women's lovers.)

Many women experience breast tenderness, heaviness, or the occasional ache. If this continues for any length of time, or if you discover anything that you feel uneasy with whilst doing your monthly breast examination, or at any other time, consult your practitioner. Every year, over 31,000 women die in the UK with breast cancer.

Cervical screening – the smear test

Some women find this very invasive. The insult to the tender cervix of repeated scraping may also contribute to difficulties in this area. It is, however, the only medical method of early detection for cervical cancer, and doctors recommend a test every three to five years. Surface changes in the cervix can be seen by inserting a speculum to hold the vaginal walls open, and looking in. This is part of what is involved in an internal examination and you can do this for yourself with the aid of a mirror. The cervix can change quite noticeably through each menstrual cycle, and regular checks will enable you to get to know the differences, and let you get used to what is normal for you.

In the medical procedure, a scraping of cells is taken from the cervix with a small spatula. These are then examined in a laboratory to see whether there are any changes in the cell structure that could point to problems, or the possibility of cancer. Results can take up to twelve weeks to reach your doctor and the test will need to be repeated if there was any insufficiency of cells, if the investigation was incomplete or if any minor changes have been noted. In the final part of any pelvic examination, the condition of your abdomen will be felt, and here the examiner is looking for any small lumps around the ovaries. This is the only real method of their early detection.

What to Eat Now

Food has traditionally been the source of great sensual pleasure. Eating some specific foods can be highly suggestive, but there is a great delight to be found in meeting any appetite. Sex is traditionally better before a meal, when there is a slight hunger, or at least when not feeling full. Some people, however, find the satisfaction of having eaten the perfect prelude to an amorous encounter. It helps if you and your lover agree on this point.

There is little proof that foods can act specifically as aphrodisiacs, although some do have reputations for increasing virility or improving sexual function. Peppermint tea, garlic, onions, cloves and spices like ginger traditionally inflame sexual passion. Myrrh is especially useful for women, rejuvenating and restoring energy to the whole reproductive system. Rose is traditionally a symbol of love, and the scent works as an effective uterine tonic. Avoiding all these, and taking some weak comfrey tea once a week may suppress sexual desire.

In general, a healthy body is a sexy body, so a good all-round diet supplemented by vitamins and minerals or herbs where necessary (at the change of season, or to meet specific health needs) is recommended. Zinc is necessary to all sexual function. It is found in animal flesh, milk and milk products, bread and cereals, and pumpkin seeds, or it can be taken as a supplement.

When it comes to overall health, a healthy heart is essential to ongoing physical prowess in every sphere of life. It is the most important aspect of ongoing healthcare. Adding oat bran to the diet, increasing the amount of water you drink, reducing the amount of animals and animal products that you eat, and increasing your intake of cold-pressed, extra-virgin olive oil will all help your heart. Reduce the level of artificial stimulants in your diet, and consider making some of the following changes:

Reduce	*Substitute*
Red meat	White meat, fish, vegetable protein, grain and pulse combinations
White sugar	Fruit, fruit juices, muscovado sugar, honey
White flour	Wholegrain flour
Wheat	Other grains: corn, oats, millet, rye, soya and potato flour
Cows' dairy produce	Goats' and ewes' milk products, soya milk, tofu, almond, rice and coconut milks
Coffee and tea	Chicory and herbal-based coffee drinks, herbal tisanes, warm fruit drinks
Salt	Herbs, fresh and dried, Gomasio
Margarine and spreads	Unsalted butter, olive oil, Vitaquell
Salad creams and mayonnaise	Cold-pressed extra-virgin

	olive oil and lemon juice dressing, whipped tofu
Peanut butters	Tahini
Stock cubes	Herbs, spices, cornmeal
MSG and preservatives	Herbs and spices

Emily first consulted me with a range of symptoms that didn't quite seem to fit together. A busy twenty-one-year-old, she felt tired a lot of the time, had a range of small, niggly skin complaints, and suffered with vaginal thrush and athlete's foot. She felt altogether uncomfortable in her body and derived little satisfaction from physical activity, and she also had little interest in food except for occasional episodes when she would go on what she called her 'sugar fest'.

She began to follow a sugar- and yeast-free diet, and within three days noticed a distinct improvement in her energy levels. She applied a honey pack to her skin complaints each night, and added a capful of apple cider vinegar to her bathwater each day to help with the thrush. Within six weeks her diet was back to near normal and she was feeling well again.

Her physical recovery was good, but she still seemed to have little connection with or interest in her body. In one session she told me that she had been celibate for two years, and admitted to feeling rather unloved and uncared for. I suggested she take a Sitz Bath (see p.90) every week, and book a massage or aromatherapy session every week too. For the next six weeks she concentrated on measures to increase her interest, and entice her energy back into her body. At her last annual check-up, she had been free from all her symptoms for six months, and was feeling much better in herself. She still takes care not to allow too much sugar or yeast in her diet, and has regular body treats.

Staying Well

- Add a capful of apple cider vinegar to bathwater at least once a week to help normalise vaginal pH. This is especially useful if thrush has been a problem, or if being sexually active.
- As a regular measure, crouch down when in the shower, and allow the water to spray directly onto the kidney region of your lower back for a few minutes. This is warming and gently stimulating, and may well encourage you to urinate. This is very useful if cystitis has been a difficulty in the past.
- I want to extol the virtues of natural methods of contraception because they are very relevant, but during these times of increasingly worrying sexually transmitted diseases, barrier methods must be given priority. These are also the kindest to the body of all medical choices, having few, if any, side effects. The worst that can happen is a localised reaction to the spermicide, and this is quite a rare thing. Compared to the devastating effects of taking the contraceptive pill, or wearing an IUD, these are definitely a good choice. The pill has a lasting impact on menstruation and fertility, and confuses the body's hormones and nutritional needs.

Natural methods of contraception can be used in combination with a condom, and preferably the practice of safer sex, for extremely good results in terms of ongoing health and protection from unplanned pregnancy. We are, after all, only actively fertile for a few days every month. As ways of getting to know your own body better, and deepening your understanding of the way your body works, these techniques are fantastic.

Most natural choices of contraception rely upon periods of abstinence from intercourse. They aim to identify changes in the cycle that can pin-point ovulation and therefore the 'riskiest' time if conception is to be avoided. Sexual appetite tends to peak at ovulation, when fertility is at its highest, and again before menstruation.

The rhythm or calendar method assumes that ovulation will occur fourteen days before menstruation and that each cycle will be of exactly the same length. All women know their cycles can be affected by relationships, sexual activity, emotional well-being, the season and a host of other factors.

The most common form of natural contraception is to combine two techniques that will pin-point fertility. This involves taking your temperature immediately on waking with a specially calibrated thermometer, and charting this along with changes in vaginal mucus. These should enable you to feel really in touch with your body's changing cycle and to see how it affects and is affected by other aspects of your life and the natural world. We commonly ovulate at one of the phases of the moon, and will experience energy changes and an emotional response too. (See Fertility, p. 131).

It is important to get to know your cycle well if you wish to use this information as the basis of contraception. It is recommended that you abstain from having sex at all for a few months to establish what is normal for you, although this too can influence the findings.

Managing stress

Women have always used our bodies as a part of our own healing. Rhythmic movement whether in dance or exercise is fundamentally important to our well-being. Dance is something we can all take pleasure in, whether it is done alone at home with the radio turned on, or in a club, as part of a group or class, or as a social ritual or celebration. It is one of the most embraceable forms of exercise because of its combination of movement and rhythm with the power of music.

Experience this for yourself by introducing some regular, harmonious, rhythmic movement into your daily routine as one of your tools for managing stress, and you will soon feel a difference in your life.

CIRCLE DANCE

Spend a few minutes every morning or evening freeing your body and allowing it to move and express itself through movement, and you will see effects within days. The first benefits are often in terms of both physical and mental suppleness and clarity of mind.

You will soon be able to discern more subtle signs and improvements – you may feel moved to laugh, or shed a tear, or be reminded of minor aches. These movement moments have a diagnostic use in terms of sensing and expressing just how happy your body is.

You can do this dancing to music or unaccompanied. It is good to focus on a type of movement to provide a framework for the mind to work within, especially at the beginning. A circle is a good symbol for fluidity and movement, and moving in a circle is a good way to start. Fix your feet flat on the floor about shoulder-width apart. This will provide a solid and secure base that will allow the rest of your body to make a lot of movement. Begin by moving your pelvis round in a slow circle. Then include your knees in the movement so the whole of your lower body is involved in the gliding, circular motion. Your upper body will naturally be ready to join in, so continue the circular theme by gently and slowly circling your head, and making circles with your hands and with your arms. Mirror the circles of your pelvis with your shoulders, and surrender to the movement, and feel the tremendous sense of energy and freedom as you glide and move through the circle of this experience.

Using a fluid, circular movement is a wonderful way to open up your body to this means of expressing itself. This is an exercise in trusting your body to do what it needs, so follow your body's lead and allow it to make whatever movements are needed. These may at times be erratic, or asymmetrical, or change in tempo or intensity – this is your body expressing itself.

Use this exercise to notice whether there are any parts of you that do not move freely, or to discover where different feelings live, or for the simple joy it will bring to your day.

Cystitis

Discomfort on urinating doesn't sound too bad, but anyone who has ever suffered with this painful and depleting condition knows just how difficult it can be. If there is blood in your urine or if you experience pain in your lower back or if you are unsure of the diagnosis, then please consult your practitioner and have this checked. They will usually take a urine test to confirm what type of infection is causing the problem.

Start drinking large amounts of water as soon as you notice a problem. Once you feel able, alternate unsweetened cranberry juice and weak chamomile tea with the water, and keep drinking large amounts. If urinating is very painful, sit in a large bowl or a shallow bath filled with warm water and it won't hurt.

As soon as you feel able to leave the comfort of the water, keep drinking, and make a warm compress to place on your abdomen, just above your pubic bone, where your pubic hair starts. Add a few drops of essential oil of Olibanum or some strong chamomile tea to a bowl of warm water, and soak a wad of cotton fabric in it. Wring out well, and place this on the abdomen surrounded and covered with a towel. Place a hot water bottle on your lower back just over your sacrum, and another between your legs. Each time you actually urinate, rinse yourself well by sitting in a bowl full of warm water, and then dab yourself dry very gently.

Keep yourself warm, and don't try and hide your feelings – cry and moan if you feel moved to. It all helps release the tension. Once recovery is in sight, take echinacea or a multivitamin supplement to reinforce your immune system and help you feel stronger. Avoid alcohol, coffee, cigarettes and spicy foods, and reduce sugar.

Personal hygiene is of fundamental importance in avoiding attacks. In the toilet, always wipe from front to back, and wash your hands after every visit. Pay scrupulous attention to gentle cleansing, and wash if possible after a bowel movement. Take care to change underwear daily, and avoid synthetic fabrics. Wear stockings rather than tights, and skirts or loose-fitting trousers. External sanitary protection is recommended, but take care to change pads regularly, and wash if possible at stages throughout the day. Do not be tempted to use fragranced soaps, feminine deodorants or perfumed wipes. Water is fine, or use with an oatmeal sack, or Ayurvedic or gentle soap. Always urinate as soon as possible after intercourse, and wash too. Cystitis can be caused by uncommon sexual activity, when the delicate area of the vulva can become bruised. This usually passes quite quickly, and will respond equally well to all the above measures.

Thrush

This is characterised by itching and soreness throughout the whole genital region, and a creamy, white vaginal discharge. It is important to ensure that this is not any other infection if you have been sexually active. Barrier methods of contraception can cause this type of response, particularly as a reaction to spermicidal gels or creams that can irritate the delicate vulva. Uncommon sexual activity can also generate these symptoms.

Treat by eliminating sugar and wheat from your diet completely for five days. Gain immediate relief by spreading some cold natural live yoghurt on a feminine pad and applying it, changing as often as required. Take frequent baths and add a capful of apple cider vinegar to the water. Wear skirts or very loose-fitting trousers, stockings instead of tights, and no knickers whenever possible. Avoid taking antibiotics, herbal alternatives often work just as well. Antibiotics usually cause havoc in the body, killing not just the desired infection, but everything else, including all the beneficial bacteria that live in our gut and are essential for full absorption of our food, and controlling *candida* overgrowth. One of the reasons for the increase in *candida* or yeast infections is the seemingly indiscriminate use of antibiotics. If you really must take them, follow each course with a supplement of B-complex vitamins, and large amounts of garlic and fresh live yoghurt or acidophilus and bifidus powder to help repopulate the gut.

If no relief is gained, douche twice daily with a teaspoon of apple cider vinegar in two pints of warm water, and wear a garlic tampon at night for three nights. To make this, carefully peel a garlic clove so as not to remove the thin membrane that covers it. Pierce the clove with a sterilised needle which has been threaded with a length of double cotton. This allows just enough of the potent garlic to escape, but not too much that could burn the vagina. Insert like a tampon, as far as you can reach with a very clean finger. Remove on waking, and douche with the apple cider vinegar mixture.

Genital warts

Visit your practitioner for specific help with combating this. In the meantime, if the warts are external, paint them carefully with Thuja tincture. This is in an alcohol base, so take care when applying, and use a cotton bud or small painting brush to aid accuracy. Ti-tree oil can also be used.

Take ten drops of echinacea tincture in water, lots of fresh garlic, and one cup of nettle tea daily, along with some propolis and aloe vera. These will all promote the body's immune system in various ways and aid detoxification or elimination of the virus.

It is important to recognise that this virus has been implicated in the incidence of cervical cancer, so if you suspect that you have it, consider taking annual smear tests and protect your cervix by always using a barrier form of contraceptive.

Genital herpes

This devastating condition will respond well to both dietary changes and local treatments, but it can take time, and developing a personal programme with your practitioner is advised.

Remove from your diet as far as possible all foods

containing large amounts of the amino acid arginine. These include cocoa, brown rice, all nuts, peas, beans, seeds, gelatine, coconut, onions, coffee and tea. Other foods contain traces but not in quantities to be harmful. Take a lysine supplement of 500mg a day. Also take 1g of vitamin C, a multivitamin and mineral supplement, ten drops of echinacea tincture in a little water and some propolis every day. This needs to be continued for about a year after the attack, so bear with it, and consult your practitioner regularly for monitoring and individual advice.

During an attack, consider simplifying your diet as much as possible in order to free up energy for the body to effect healing. Switch to eating rice and lightly steamed vegetables or vegetable broth, or freshly extracted vegetable juices. Drink large amounts of water and stay warm. Keep your feet warm especially, and let your emotions flow.

Caroline first came to see me looking for general help. She had a history of pelvic problems, including endometriosis, and had also contracted herpes which was having a devastating effect. A slight woman in her early 30s, she was experiencing herpes attacks every month, with her period, and looked very weak. A blood test confirmed that she was anaemic.

She began taking a daily dose of the amino acid lysine, along with large amounts of vitamin C, a protein powder, and a multivitamin and mineral capsule. She applied neat Ti-tree oil to the herpes blisters when they appeared, and modified her diet to include large amounts of garlic and ginger, and a variety of good sources of iron. She also took twenty drops of echinacea tincture twice a day.

Within two months she was noticeably stronger, and her iron levels were improving. She was able to feel better in herself, and her periods were becoming less painful. After a series of monitored fasts, during which she ate only fruit and drank lots of water, her body was recovering ground, and the herpes attacks, although continuing, occurred only once over three months.

At her six-month check-up, she had been able to start a new job, move house and begin a new relationship – all things she had not before felt strong enough to even contemplate. Her health was continuing to improve, and she maintained her high level of supplementation until, as she put it, 'all is absolutely 100 per cent'.

Vaginal infections

A wide range of vaginal infections can occur, all with similar symptoms. Visit your practitioner for an accurate diagnosis, and in the meantime treat symptomatically. A poultice made from powdered slippery elm mixed with cool water can be placed on a sanitary pad and applied to the whole area to soothe and cool any irritation. Use a garlic tampon (see p.127) immediately any problem occurs, and add one capful of apple cider vinegar to bath water. Take echinacea and myrrh either as tinctures (ten drops in a little water twice a day) or as one cup of each tea every day. These will stimulate the immune system and help fight the infection. Supplement your diet with 1g of vitamin C with each meal.

Take 4oz (110g) of calendula and soak in a saucepan containing about four pints (2,300ml) of water overnight. In the morning, bring the pot to the boil, and then strain the liquid into a bath full of water. Soak in the bath for at least twenty minutes, making sure that the level of the water reaches up over your kidneys. Do not use any soap. Pat dry gently, and sit for at least ten minutes, wrapped up in towels to rest before doing anything else. If you have experienced any backache, or are feeling particularly fearful or uneasy, make with a mixture of 2oz (55g) calendula and 2oz (55g) yarrow.

Make sure that you allow lots of air to circulate between your legs, so consider not wearing any underwear whenever possible, and choose skirts rather than trousers, cotton knickers rather than synthetic fabrics, and stockings rather than tights.

Resources

The Tao of Love and Sex Jolan Chan, Wildwood House Press
Kitty Campion's Handbook of Herbal Health Kitty Campion, Sphere
How to Stay Out of the Gynecologist's Office Federation of Feminist Women's Health Centres, Women to Women (USA)
Breast Cancer Care 26A Harrison Street, London WC1H 8JG. 0171 867 1103
Rape Crisis Centre PO Box 69, London WC1. 0171 837 1600
Institute of Psychosexual Medicine Cavendish Square, 11 Chandos Street, London W1M 9DE. 0171 580 0631

FERTILITY

With every monthly cycle we experience the opportunity of fertility. The twin peak of energy that balances the menstrual flow is ovulation, the time when a new egg begins its journey of possibility, and our fertility is reaffirmed. Around fourteen days after the start of each period, an egg is made ready to leave one of the ovaries and journey down the fallopian tube to reach the uterus. This whole procedure is orchestrated by the hormones circulating in the system in response to the work of the pituitary gland in the brain. The next two days are the key time when sperm is likely to meet the egg in the fallopian tube if fertilisation is to occur. Over the next three days or so, the egg will continue its journey down to the uterus, and after about another two days will safely embed itself there. If fertilised, the process of cell division will already have begun, and the woman is unlikely to have her next period.

The exact timing of each event in the cycle may vary, and some months may pass without ovulation, or one ovary may be more active than the other. When fertility is being courted, these details become enormously important in the quest for the perfect moment to conceive.

Nowadays more women are choosing to conceive later in life, perhaps after starting a career, or when more financially stable and emotionally mature. After the age of thirty-five, our fertility really takes a nosedive (this is often due to the steady decline in nutritional states that tends to hit us at this age), and additional measures may be necessary to encourage conception. Today we are also seeing many women choosing artificial insemination as a route to achieving a pregnancy.

A growing number of women choose not to have children, preferring to express their creative energy in other ways. These women need to actively take time out for themselves, to reassess their career, their life structure, etc., because they do not have the automatic break or breaks that pregnancy can afford. It is also vital to ensure that their creativity is used to the full in whatever other areas they channel their energy.

Infertility is an increasing problem. As our lives become more distanced from the natural world and the toxins in our environment increase, it is our sensitive reproductive systems that bear the brunt of this assault. Potentially toxic factors as wide ranging as computer and TV screen emissions to food dyes seem to impact upon our lives in ever-increasing ways. Sitting too close to a TV screen (less than six feet away) depletes vitamin A stores in the body. Male computer screen workers have been proven to have noticeably lower sperm counts than normal, and there is a suspicion that the same deleterious effects are wreaking havoc on women's bodies.

The chemicals from intensive farming have leaked into the water table, and we can now take in large quantities of pesticides with each glass of milk. These are the same pesticides that cause infertility in other mammals. Our sedentary lifestyle also has an impact on the health of the pelvis. When fat stores accumulate around the reproductive organs, they have a physical restricting effect, as well as drawing toxins to the site (heavy metals, chemicals, etc. are all stored in fat cells). Use it or lose it seems to fit here, because regular sexual activity increases blood flow to the whole pelvic region and is one of the nicest health-promoting measures I can suggest.

Spending some time simplifying life and getting back in touch with our instinctive senses is always the first step in redressing any imbalance and restoring our fertility. It is important to avoid the artificial, from situations and emotions to foods and fabrics.

Managing Change

What a rich learning ground this area is. We spend much of our lives blocking our fertility, or anxiously cultivating it. What a shock it can be when after years of taking steps to stop conception, we find that it is not an automatic event.

This is especially the case for women who decide to have children later in life. At one time, girls who had babies before they were twenty were really considered silly, and everyone thought it made sense to wait until we had done other things with our lives. Those other things, especially careers, can take a long time. Now women are choosing to have their first baby in their thirties and forties. By then, our eggs, like our bodies, are getting older, and conception is not guaranteed.

It is a shock when we don't conceive, and it opens the door for a whole range of negative emotions from self-doubt to anger. Every menstrual period can become a sad reminder of a very personal failure. For women who may have achieved so much in their lives, this can be a very difficult mountain to climb.

There are wonderful opportunities here to discover our own inner child, and to bring more love into our own lives. A whole branch of therapy is devoted to this, and many counselling techniques seek to develop our relationship with our own inner child. It is a powerful way to both understand and heal the pains of the past, and also develops any areas of ourself that are in need of nurturing and care. We also enhance the ability of our own inner parent, and this has a wonderfully positive effect on our lives.

It is wonderful to let go of the weight of adult responsibilities and worries and release that youthful joy and exuberance. Begin by thinking of all the things you imagine being able to do with your child, then do them with yourself. Go carol singing, build that go-cart, learn children's songs, feed the ducks in the park, learn another language, start finger painting, etc. Another good idea is to give your 'child' anything that she wanted when she was little, but couldn't have. This might be time, and care, and lots of cuddles, or it might be a box of Lego and some dance classes.

Expressing creativity

Creativity is an energy that is present throughout life, and it is worth exploring the many different ways that you have to channel it. Having a baby is one very definite way of expressing creative energy. It is a good idea not to restrict our creativity to one sole expression, but rather to explore the richness of available avenues and forms, knowing that opening oneself in this way never depletes, but rather allows more creativity to flow.

When creative energy is blocked or suppressed, the feelings of frustration and impotence can spill into other areas of life, upsetting general health and equilibrium. Using creative energy in any positive way has a balancing effect for the whole person.

There are many ways in which we can express our creativity on a daily basis, even though we may not all be able to produce beautiful works of art or a literary masterpiece.

Keeping a daily journal is a creative way to work with

your feelings and emotions; it's fun to play with paints and colour if it attracts you, and creating beauty and order within the home or immediate environment can be deeply satisfying. Expressing yourself creatively, through music, singing, or any form of craft work is wonderful.

Gardening is an especially creative pursuit and can be enjoyed indoors, in window boxes, and on terraces and allotments if a garden is not available. Creating good nourishment for ourselves and expressing love through it is a wonderfully rewarding activity, whether this is in fact a tasty meal or the gift of time to spend enjoying or relaxing at the end of a busy day.

Your Body Now

With the spotlight on fertility, it is possible to lose sight of the rest of our experience, and total body care is essential for ongoing full health. Although it is important to focus on goals and desires, being in touch with our bodies, and at ease with our own physicality, is an excellent start for any project. It is also one of the great gifts that we can pass on to our children by example.

Now is the time to explore some of the ways that you can foster feelings of physical integrity and pleasure. Consider anything that unites your experience – your own ideas will inevitably be most appropriate, but massage, exercise and meditation are all a good idea. An all-over massage from a professional therapist, or even an enthusiastic lover or friend, is a wonderful way to involve the whole body and connect it all together. Physical movement, especially any that is rhythmic or to music, unites the different parts of the body in an especially potent way. If dance or aerobic classes do not interest you, what about weight training, running or walking?

Meditation is a special way of putting back all the pieces. It can be a cohesive force that will maintain you through all sorts of situations that modern life can seem to throw at you. Some people find that they are able to do this quite naturally and easily, and for others there are many training courses available. Regular meditation is a wonderful discipline to cultivate, and the positive effects will become apparent in your life as well as in your body remarkably quickly.

Cold water paddling is a wonderful and easy technique that will boost your energy levels and directly influence your circulation – which runs through your whole body, communicating between all areas and all levels of experience. Early morning cold water paddling will wake up your whole system, boosting the circulation through your pelvis and from your head to your toes. It is a marvellous way to start the day, every day.

COLD WATER PADDLING

Fill the bath about ⅓ full with cold water and step in. The water should come up well over your ankles. If a bath is not available use a large washing-up bowl or a baby bath. Walk up and down in the water for about a minute, then step out and sit down on a chair or the side of the bath for a few moments. You will probably already begin to feel the benefits of a clearer head and warm, toasty feet.

What to Eat Now

Eating well is an important tool in maintaining full health, and more so when preparing for pregnancy, which takes its toll on the body's reserves. The first step, though, is to cleanse the system, so that any toxins can be removed, along with potential blocks to full absorption, assimilation and digestion. With toxins playing such a vital role in the dysfunction of the whole body, it is vital to cleanse the system as much as possible as a first step towards heightening fertility.

Begin by introducing fast days into your normal routine. this will be one day each week, or each month, when you plan to give your digestive system a complete break. When you are continuously processing, digesting and assimilating foods you are actually using quite a lot of energy. By simplifying the job of digestion and making life easier on the body, all that energy is freed up to get on with other work within the body. The first job is most usually to detoxify the system.

One of the simplest forms of detox is to choose one fruit or vegetable, and to eat only that for the day, along with drinking plenty of water. Apples, pears, grapes, carrots and celery are all excellent choices, and you can eat as much of any one of them as you please. If you prefer, you can substitute freshly extracted juices, but make sure you 'chew' the juice a little before swallowing. Juice fasts are an excellent way to ensure large amounts of quality vitamins and minerals.

Once used to this system, you can begin to introduce fast days as a response to health concerns, so when you get a cold, or hurt your back, or suffer with ovulation pains, switch your body into cleansing mode by following a day's fast.

Your whole diet can become more cleansing by focusing on different foods. Garlic is a natural antibiotic and can be included on a daily basis. Mung beans and rice are both easily digested, and excellent for carrying toxins out of the system. These can easily form a major part of your diet. Raw or very lightly steamed foods can be excellent sources of fibre as well as providing necessary nutrients. Avoid chemical additives and all foods that contain them, including MSG and other artificial flavourings, colourings and adulterants. Become scrupulous about the quality of your food and consider the benefits of naturally grown fruit and vegetables over those that are chemically treated.

Limit the amount of animal flesh and animal products that you consume, including cows' dairy produce. (A recent Government survey showed that industrial pesticides had been found in 50 per cent of the commercially available cows' milk that they tested. High levels of one in particular had been the cause of infertility in other mammals.)

Consider following a raw diet for three days each month, preferably around ovulation time. Plan to eat only raw foods and drink plenty of water. (During the winter months, add some cooked rice, and some paprika, cinnamon, cloves or chillies for warmth, and drink some hot water and herbal teas.)

Consult your practitioner for further monitored detoxification, or follow the detailed directions in *The Detox Diet Book*.

Ensure good levels of vitamins and minerals in your diet, and consider supplementing with zinc, vitamin B12, and 1g of vitamin C each day. Manganese is also essential to fertility, so ensure its presence in your multivitamin and mineral supplement, along with selenium and vitamin E.

Staying Well

- Sunlight is a nutrient in itself and its effect on the brain will help regulate all the body's natural cycles. Spending some time out in natural light every day will have a positive effect on the system. I have known this simple 'cure' to rebalance a woman's cycles within as little as one month.

Make sure to spend at least twenty minutes every day out-doors without wearing sun-glasses – the sunlight needs to touch the eyes, but, as always, never look directly into the sun. This is most effective during the warmer months, but the same effect can be gained if you stay outdoors for longer during the winter months. But remember that we have done so much damage to our earth's own protective systems that it is no longer safe to go out into the sun as freely as we used to. Take great care to limit your sun exposure to times of day when the sun's rays are least damaging: never go out in the middle of the day without good protection. You are looking for the benefit of the *light*, and this can be received in the early morning and late afternoon.

- Natural forms of birth control all focus on pin-pointing ovulation as accurately as possible. This makes them potentially wonderful aids to conception. The most well-known of these methods, the Rhythm or Calendar method, is a rather hit and miss affair that depends upon ovulation occurring each month fourteen days after the start of the last period. This is a good starting point in that at least it puts us in the right part of the cycle.

The Temperature method involves keeping a specially cali-brated thermometer (available from your pharmacist) by your bed, and taking your temperature the moment you wake every morning. The thermometer will record tiny degrees of change, and if you record them regularly, you should start to see a pattern emerge after a few months.

This takes some care, because the degree of difference is

so small. Essentially, the resting temperature will be very slightly raised at the time of ovulation. It is marked by a rise in the basal body temperature of about 0.6–0.8 of a degree. If you chart the temperature through the month you should be able to pin-point ovulation at about the midpoint of this rise in temperature, between the start of the increase and its peak. In combination with mucus testing, this can give you quite accurate results.

Mucus testing involves quite simply testing vaginal mucus every day immediately after taking your temperature. You are actually testing for the secretions from the cervix, so slip your finger into your vagina, and when you remove it, see how sticky it is. This will change enormously through each cycle, ranging from being watery and clear, becoming much more profuse and having an elastic quality around the time of ovulation.

An egg will live between six and twenty-four hours after ovulation. If the woman's mucus is a good environment, sperm may live for up to five days in it. There is, therefore, a potential seven-day period in each cycle when fertilisation is possible.

At the end of each menstrual period, there is little mucus. You feel dry and there is no mucus evidence on underwear. About six days before ovulation is due, mucus appears that is quite thin, clear, slippery and runny (like a raw egg white). As ovulation occurs this becomes more elastic or stretchy. Immediately after ovulation, as the 'window' closes, the mucus will become rather sticky as opposed to slippery and lose all its elasticity. It then becomes opaque rather than clear, and may leave the familiar lightly coloured mark on underwear.

Obviously, to follow all of these measures requires a degree of dedication, especially initially when you are coming to recognise the changes in your own cycle, and what is

Anne wanted to improve her overall health, and consulted me with fertility as a secondary matter – she was considering planning a family in the coming year. We discussed a few dietary changes and some physical, exercise routines to tone up her body, but her imagination was not captured. She was twenty-eight and a busy manager who admitted to being stressed most of the time, and needed to feel really fuelled by a thing in order to pursue it.

So we made her health into a project. She was given homework tasks to complete between each appointment, and these began with organising her life into areas of well-being and imbalance. She came back with a card file which she had filled with different areas of her health and lifestyle that she could identify, and we worked to identify goals and challenges within each section.

It soon became clear that she wanted a baby very much indeed, and we set about planning an organised campaign of action to achieve that goal. She was the most dedicated person I had ever seen, and achieved almost every goal she set herself, from clearing out the house and making a nursery corner in their bedroom, to detoxifying her body, and clearing her mind. The card file was her way of focusing on the project, and she was able to identify all that she needed to do. She attended a class in child development alongside learning about the latest moves in nutrition. She had been charting her fertility with great care, and she and her husband were having great fun with the project. At her last appointment she was three months pregnant, and blissfully happy.

normal for you. It is remarkably easy though to begin to pay attention to your changing mucus levels, and to watch for energy and temperature changes that accompany them. If you are going to chart your cycle (see p.142) it is recommended that you abstain from sexual activity, and this will enable you

FERTILITY AWARENESS CHART

Date: 5th January : (Day One Of Cycle)

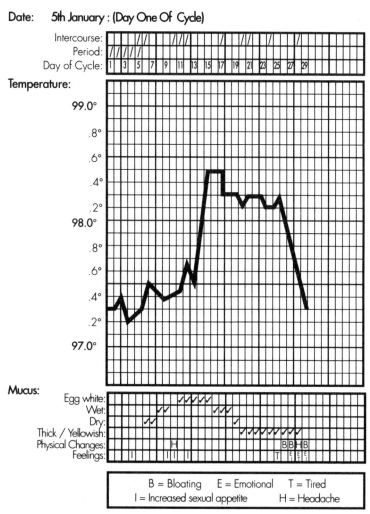

B = Bloating   E = Emotional   T = Tired
I = Increased sexual appetite   H = Headache

FERTILITY AWARENESS CHART

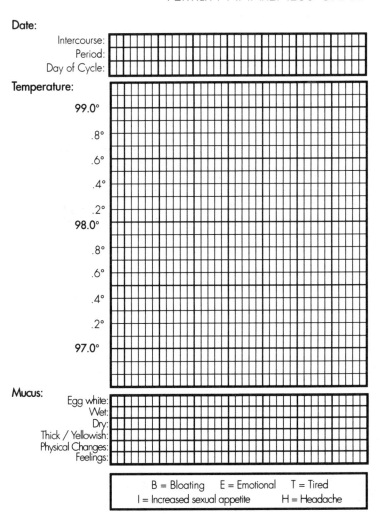

Date:
Intercourse:
Period:
Day of Cycle:
Temperature:
99.0°
.8°
.6°
.4°
.2°
98.0°
.8°
.6°
.4°
.2°
97.0°
Mucus:
Egg white:
Wet:
Dry:
Thick / Yellowish:
Physical Changes:
Feelings:

B = Bloating   E = Emotional   T = Tired
I = Increased sexual appetite   H = Headache

to chart your own changes more fully and accurately. There are now machines on the market that will pin-point your fertile time by analysing a small sample of your urine. These can be used safely at home, and are a useful and effective tool. The process of getting to know your body, though, is one that you can still continue even with the machine as back-up.

Managing stress

External stresses become internal stresses when they impact upon our lives in an unwelcome way. Holding tension in the body is a terrible habit which reduces blood flow and therefore inhibits proper function. We have a tendency today to live much more sedentary lifestyles than our forebears, and this too can add to pelvic congestion and other areas of tension.

RELAXING

Physical relaxation is a very useful technique to learn, because as well as being totally relaxing for the whole body, it can also be used to spotlight a specific area. You can also do this just about anywhere.

Make yourself comfortable in a chair with your feet flat on the floor. Take off your shoes and loosen any tight or restricting clothing. Take a few deep, cleansing breaths right down into your belly and imagine yourself settling and becoming a little more relaxed as your limbs become a little heavier and you let go of any tensions. You are going to learn how to recognise and then release physical stresses. If it is easier for you to do this lying down, place a pillow under your knees and another to support your neck, this will keep your back as relaxed as possible. There is a temptation to fall asleep as you relax more and more deeply, and if this happens you may wish to do the exercise in two parts, starting again where you left off whenever you wake.

Begin with your left foot, and clench in the toes as you breathe in, holding them tight as you breathe out. Squeeze hard. Breathe in again, and this time let your toes uncurl and relax as you breathe out. Take a breath and enjoy the feeling in your toes. Then tighten up your whole foot as you breathe in, holding it tight as you breathe out. Squeeze hard. Breathe in again, and this time let your foot relax as you breathe out. Take a breath and enjoy the feeling in your foot.

Continue this pattern up your left leg and hip, then from your right foot up to your left hip, then clench and relax your bottom, your tummy, and all the way up your body to your shoulders. Clench and relax first your left hand and arm, and then your right, and continue on up, working your neck, your face, and your hair-line.

Finish by returning to your feet and breathing some deep, cleansing breaths as you clench and then relax both feet together. Sit still for a few minutes, continuing the gentle breathing, and enjoy the feelings in your body.

Repeat this daily. At first it will take quite some time to work your way through the whole body, but you will soon find your own trouble spots and be able to tailor to exercise to suit your own patterns of tension. Once you are confident, extend the exercise to include relaxing your organs and glands as well by working on an inner smile. Picture your whole body smiling, inside. Begin with your pineal gland in the middle of your forehead, and carry on down through your eyes, your tonsils, your stomach, diaphragm, etc., to your womb. Picture them all in turn smiling – gently relaxing, curling up, and letting go. Finish with some easy, relaxed breaths, and an external smile.

Pre-conceptual care

This is one of the best ways of preparing yourself for parenthood, as well as enhancing the health of prospective children. The genetic information that we pass on is like a blueprint for all their future growth and development. The mother's immunity is passed directly to the baby with early breast milk, and the lifestyle patterns we live will serve as a model to our children for the whole of their lives.

A positive model of health consciousness is one of the best parental gifts. This means that well before the pregnancy is the time to be taking regular exercise, become more conscious of good nutrition, schedule rest and play into the routine, and make whatever changes are needed to redress any imbalances, and provide for a healthy future for the whole family.

Ideally, both parents could prepare themselves for conception over the preceding year. This allows time for the whole body to get ready, and pass on the best possible health future to their child.

As soon as you begin thinking about conception:

- Stop smoking and drinking alcohol. Apart from their terrible effects on the body, you will soon be a role model for a young innocent child who needs to learn good health habits from you.
- Switch to barrier methods of contraception. This will give your body time to cleanse itself if you have been taking the pill, or using an IUD, and for your hormones to rebalance.
- Avoid X-rays and heavy pollution. They both take their toll on the body through requiring so much work internally to repair the damage or cope with the problem.

This is energy that you want to use in other ways.

- Stop using aluminium cooking utensils. You do not need this metal in the amounts that you will be exposed to if you cook all your meals in it. Studies have implicated it in cases of severe impairment of the body's normal functioning when traces are accumulated over a lifetime's exposure.
- Learn ways to relax and manage your stress levels. These are good health habits that will prolong your life and improve its quality.
- Instigate an exercise programme to improve your all-round fitness and stamina.
- Learn all you can about nutrition – both for your own sake, because pregnancy is hard work for the body, and so that you will be able to provide your child with the best nutrients.
- Consult a naturopath or other practitioner for a full health assessment. This will enable you to redress any particular health concerns prior to pregnancy, and will establish a relationship that can guide you through the coming years.
- Set to work improving your constitution, taking whatever dietary supplements are necessary for your own optimum health.
- Consider learning about or taking a class in child development and parenting skills. These will help you prepare for a child, and focus your energy on your goal.

Remember that if you are successful, that moment will remain forever in your memory and in the imagination of your child, so make each attempt as good as it can possibly be in every respect. If you regularly reach orgasm the whole area is likely to have a better tone, although it is not necessary to orgasm in order to conceive.

Infertility

Many couples do not conceive as quickly as they would like. If you do find you are having difficulty, consider the measures outlined in the text for cleansing your diet and your lifestyle. Herbal remedies may help strengthen and reinforce the work of your hormonal and reproductive systems, and you should consult your practitioner for individual guidance.

The power of our desires is phenomenal, and when we unite all our energies and focus ourselves on a particular outcome, the effect can be awesome. The power of the mind is not to be ignored when wanting some physical outcome, and positive thought, affirmations, repetitive chant and visualisation are all effective techniques that can reinforce your intentions at this time. Spend some time every day focusing on your desire – daydream about it, or paint or imagine what it will be like. Make your own personal affirmation that you can repeat to yourself throughout the day, or write down and read it aloud to yourself or with your partner.

Remember, too, that fertility can be seen as part of a bigger picture. If you have any spiritual understanding it may guide you at this time. Although the religions that cultivate guilt may not be much assistance, any true spirituality will support you in your efforts to conceive, and offer a framework for understanding what is happening whether you are successful or not. When facing difficulties, consider the possibility that this is an event you may have chosen, that you may not be ready to be the kind of parent that your child needs, or that the time may not yet be right. Whatever the reason, facing the situation with as much courage as you can find enriches you in many ways.

Resources

Yin Yang Cookbook Oliver and Michele Cowmeadow, Optima

Getting Pregnant Robert Winston, Pan

The Detox Diet Book Belinda Grant, Optima

Foresight (Association for the Promotion of Pre-conceptual Care) 28 The Paddock, Godalming, Surrey GU7 1XD. 01483 427839

Family Planning Association 27–35 Mortimer Street, London W1N 7RJ. 0171 636 7866

PREGNANCY

Pregnancy typically lasts for thirty-eight weeks, or forty weeks from the date of the last period, which is often the most accurate reference. During the first three months, the most noticeable signs will be an absence of menstruation, although some women know the moment they conceive. Each woman's body seems to respond in a different way, and no two pregnancies necessarily follow the same course. Tiredness is common in the early stages, some women experience morning sickness, breast tenderness, and an increasingly frequent need to urinate. Others will notice strange moods, or periods of reflection. Food cravings, a general happiness and changes in libido are also common. Psychics and other healers speak of the spirit or the soul entering the foetus at around the twelfth week. Usually by then most women have had their pregnancy confirmed.

Months four to six, the second trimester, see the foetus grow rapidly, and physical changes in the woman become more obvious. This is when the bump becomes clearly visible, breasts enlarge, nipples darken, and any earlier nausea and other unpleasant symptoms disappear. This is often accompanied by feelings of tremendous 'wellness' and increased energy levels. By the twenty-second week, most women have been aware of foetal movement, and this is called the quickening. Besides the bump being visible, many women simply glow by this point in their pregnancy; their skin gleams with health, and their hair and nails appear stronger and thicker. Movement is still easy, and many speak of feeling on top of the world.

The final three months can see a woman becoming more tired and heavy, and ready to give birth. Stretch marks may appear as the body becomes larger, and digestion changes as the stomach and the whole gut become somewhat squashed. Urination may again become frequent as the weight drops into the lower abdomen, and this draws forward on the spine resulting in possible muscle soreness or low-back pain. It is for many women a time of feeling most in touch with the prospective child, and these physical symptoms can seem of little importance compared to the magnitude of the event itself.

Anna was forty-two years old and had worked with me for about a year to improve her overall health. She came to see me again when she was three months pregnant with her first child, and wanted to get some advice on making the most of this time.

I made a few different suggestions including that she join a class to prepare her body for the birth. This was the one thing that she found most useful – she said it gave her a real focus, enabled her to meet other prospective mums and, most important of all, encouraged her to 'make friends with, and get to know her baby-to-be'.

She said that the habit of taking some time every day to stop and chat with the bump was wonderful, and completely changed the focus of her experience. Instead of feeling alone and a little frightened of the birth, she was able to relax into the relationship and know that they would both be involved in the whole process.

Managing Change

This can be one of the most delicious lifetime experiences, although it does take its toll on the body and is probably one of the hardest physical jobs that most women will ever undertake. Often both the bliss and the difficulty are experienced very close together, and this can characterise the event and the many ways that it will impact upon the woman's future.

It is essential that you regularly find time for yourself throughout and beyond the pregnancy. It is all too easy to become 'an expectant mother' rather than the person you have always been, and you can support your own feelings and identity best by scheduling time every week at least when you do nothing that is in any way connected with your pregnancy.

Pregnancy affords us the perfect opportunity to re-examine our relationships with our own mothers. The pregnancy is likely to deepen your connection with her, and it is easier for everyone concerned if this is as pleasurable and beneficial an experience as possible. When we are still troubled by unresolved feelings or issues around the quality of our own mothering it can get in the way of our expressing our love freely for our own children.

WRITE A LETTER TO YOUR MOTHER

One excellent way to begin to address this is to write a letter addressed to your mother. You can do this if your mother is alive or not, or whether you see her every day or not. Few mother–daughter relationships are lucky enough to allow complete openness, and there are often at least some things that you would like to say if you could speak honestly. On the other hand, this may be quite a daunting prospect, but it is remarkable what comes out once you start with a clean piece of paper and write Dear Mum at the top.

This is not a letter that you will ever send to your mother, but it is an opportunity for you to express your feelings. It may be that you could finish it in one sitting, or you may choose to put it away somewhere safe, and go back and finish it at a later date. It is a good idea for this to be as comprehensive as you can make it, so that you say all that you want to. It doesn't have to be all difficult stuff that you write, either. Sometimes the hardest things to say to our mothers are that we love them, and still need them.

There is a terrific feeling of lightness and clarity to be found in finishing such a letter. Sometimes it can be the release of words and feelings that have been unexpressed for many years.

When your letter is finished, you have a wide choice of options for what to do with it. I think it is a good idea not to keep it – you have kept the feelings, and it is good to transform this in some way. Consider committing it to a body of water that will carry it away, or tearing it into tiny pieces and letting the wind blow if out of your life. You could give it to the transforming power of fire, or dig a small hole and bury it somewhere that you then forget about, and let the earth take care of it.

The issues that writing this letter will have brought up for you can be addressed in any number of ways. You might like to raise some of them with your mother, or indeed write to her about it. Sometimes just touching on the subject can be enough to heal, and having cleared the issues for yourself, your relationship with your mother will have changed noticeably. It is good to remember that all relationships can change and grow as the partners within it change and grow. Even if some aspects remain fixed, you will have achieved a major piece of work by addressing this matter.

Your Body Now

Pregnancy, as well as being blissful, can cause considerable physical stress. It is important to understand what is happening to your body in order to make this the best possible time for you both. Dealing with all the changes can seem a little daunting, but remember what is occurring, and allow yourself to take part in the miracle. Be kind to yourself. Schedule some time every day to connect with the truth of this experience, and also to spend some time in the natural world where the whole process will seem more of a normal event. Make a point of talking to the bump, and holding and hugging it in a loving way.

Be active. Swimming, walking, and gentle hill climbing are all good exercise. You might also consider some form of gentle stretching or energy exercise such as Yoga or T'ai Chi.

Spend some time each day squatting. You can do almost anything while you are in that position, from gardening to reading, watching TV, or preparing food. This starts to stretch and open the pelvis, and releases the lower back. It is a wonderful position to cultivate feeling easy in, and may even be one of the positions you choose to give birth in. As the bump grows, you will find that your knees are pushed further apart, and this will gently stretch the hip area, and the hamstrings. If you are not used to squatting, it is not unusual to feel as though you have had quite a workout after staying in that position for any length of time. This improves with practice. If you find it difficult to begin with, support yourself by keeping your back to a wall until your legs can manage.

This is an excellent exercise for improving flexibility and loosening the whole pelvis. Do this every day, and take care to perform the exercise slowly and carefully. The aim is to achieve the gentlest of stretches, building every day over the coming months to a dramatic change.

Sit on the floor facing a clear wall. Open your legs as far as you comfortably can, without straining in any way. Shuffle carefully forwards towards the wall so that your feet are now touching it, and sit up as straight as you can, reaching forwards towards the wall with your outstretched hands. You should feel a very gentle stretch along the back of your legs and the inside of your thighs. Do not bounce, or aim to feel any discomfort, this is a soft and gentle exercise that will build over time to give you the desired results.

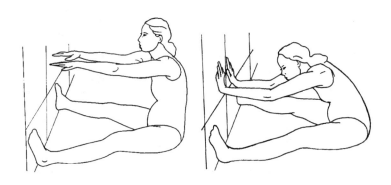

If you feel comfortable, you can move your feet a little way further apart, move your body in towards the wall so that your feet are again coming flat against it, and repeat the stretch by reaching gently forward with your upper body. Repeat this a few times in each position, and if you can feel a gentle stretching, then you have completed your exercise for today. Chart your progress weekly and you will see tremendous progress. Once you reach the stage where your hands are pressing flat against the wall, you will be able to feel the stretch by simply rocking forward slightly with your pelvis, as though you were still aiming to reach forward.

Always finish the exercise by bringing your heels together as close to your bottom as you can, and letting your knees fall out towards the floor. Then stretch your legs comfortably out in front of you with your heels flat on the floor, and 'shake out' any tension by letting your legs roll inwards and outwards in a loose rhythmic movement. This will relax all the muscles that you have been working.

What to Eat Now

Weight gain during pregnancy can vary, with the bulk of it occurring during the last twenty weeks. Appetite increases and the way you eat will alter as the pregnancy progresses, moving towards smaller, more frequent meals and a slightly lower carbohydrate content. It is so very important to eat the highest quality, purest foods available.

All fruits and vegetables are good for you. The following are high in vitamin A, C and fibre:

Vegetables: broccoli, Brussels sprouts, cabbage, carrots, cauliflower, celery, corn, courgette, cucumber, parsnip, peppers, potato, pumpkin, squash, swede, sweet potato, turnip

Fruits: apple, apricot, avocado, banana, grape, grapefruit, kiwi, mango, orange, papaya, peach, all summer berries.

Make sure fresh fruit and vegetables are always top of your shopping list, and choose lots of different kinds.

Fresh fruits and vegetables can easily be added to your existing diet:

Breakfast choices
* Start the meal with a freshly squeezed, diluted juice, fresh fruit salad or dried fruit compote
* Add banana, apple or other chopped fruit to your cereal
* Mushrooms on toast
* Add onion or tomato to scrambled eggs
* Mash banana onto toast or pancakes

Lunchtime choices
* Have a freshly extracted fruit or vegetable juice as or with the meal
* Eat at least one salad vegetable in every sandwich, e.g. lettuce, cucumber, shredded cabbage
* Fill pitta bread with mixed, dressed salad
* Choose a piece of fruit to finish the meal

Snacks
* A piece of fruit is a natural, ready-packed snack meal
* Dried fruit
* Nuts and roasted seeds
* Mixed crudités and salad leaves
* Freshly extracted juice

Dinner choices
- Corn on the cob or melon as a starter
- Salad course of a full variety of different fruits and vegetables
- Apple or other fruit in yoghurt or fromage frais
- Stewed fruit
- Fresh berries

Follow the seasons and choose fresh, locally grown produce whenever possible.

Eat regularly, and even more healthily than before. Add freshly extracted vegetable juices to your diet, and as pregnancy progresses substitute a fresh juice for a meal whenever eating becomes difficult. Find out about a balanced diet that will meet both your needs through this time. Protein is an essential, and 75g in separate helpings a day is a good target. Try to vary the diet as much as possible, so learn about combining pulses and grains to provide a complete protein, as well as having some fish, soya protein and white meat if you take it.

Calcium needs a rocket in the final three months of pregnancy. Good sources are oats, millet, sesame seeds and their products (halva, tahini and Gomasio) and raw vegetables. Iron is important throughout and again needs will increase during the final two months before labour. Good dietary sources of iron are egg yolk, molasses, soya beans, whole grains, green vegetables, fish, dried fruits, parsley, dandelion leaves, elderberries and coriander leaf (cilantro).

Include iodine at least three times a week in the form of kelp, nori and other sea vegetables and seaweeds. Zinc, magnesium, phosphorus, and vitamins A, B-complex, C, E, K (this is not often mentioned, see p.26), and folic acid are all needed and can be taken as a supplement. Folic acid is one of the B-complex vitamins and is essential during pregnancy. It is found in green leafy vegetables, brewer's yeast, beans, bananas, peas and nuts, and 400mcg every day will protect against spina bifida in your child. Specially designed pregnancy and pre-pregnancy packs with the right balance of nutrients are available from your practitioner or nutritional suppliers.

Pregnant women are medically considered to be an 'at-risk' group who need to take extra care with food preparation, handling and choice. Salmonella and listeria can both cause quite serious problems. The healthier you are generally, the least likely it is that you will suffer with any special difficulties, but take care with unpasteurised milk, soft cheeses and ice-creams, all pâtés and pre-cooked foods, especially chicken. You also need to avoid raw and undercooked eggs, and foods that contain them, e.g. mayonnaise and soufflés.

Smoking, drinking alcohol and taking any drugs at all will be potential hazards to the health of both woman and foetus.

Staying Well

- Prepare the perineum by applying ghee or sesame oil regularly after the third month. Start oiling your skin at about this time too, both as a treat for yourself, and to ward off the possibility of stretch marks. Make a massage oil by mixing almond or sesame oil, adding five drops of vitamin E oil and add one drop of essential oil of Jasmine.
- Soak a cup of calendula flowers in a tightly sealed bottle of wheatgerm or soya oil and leave for about three weeks. This makes a wonderfully soothing skin oil which can be used in conjunction with the aromatherapy mix above. Make the mixture when the moon is waxing or growing, and feel the energy of the moon's cycle reinforcing your intention.

Managing stress

There are many physical stresses involved in pregnancy, and learning to relax is vital. One of the most pleasurable ways is through the use of visualisations. Our imagination is a remarkably able and under-utilised facility that will really come into its own in protecting or assisting the body in this way. It is a lovely way to let the mind work with the body, and to unite them in one purpose that will bring harmony to the whole person.

Take some time every day to relax. Choose a quiet spot out in nature, a comfortable chair, or lying in bed first thing in the morning or for a siesta. Begin by taking a few deep, relaxing breaths, and as you breathe out imagine any tension or tightness leaving your body. Aim to clear your mind as much as possible. There are many techniques for doing this, and an easy way is to picture in your mind's eye a large cinema screen. See it in full detail, with curtains that draw in front of it and the addition of a distinct on/off switch at a point on the side. While you focus on this image there is less capacity to be seduced by other thoughts and ideas.

Once your personal cinema is clear and distinct as an image in your mind, 'hear' the music, draw back the curtains, and press the on switch. On the screen in front of you you are going to run a series of images from the natural world that will relax, inspire and rejuvenate you.

These could be memories of a wildlife documentary, images that you recall from walks or travels, or an imagined journey through a known landscape. You can choose a wood, a waterfall, valleys, mountains, the seaside . . . whatever you like. Make it as true to life as possible, and keep the image constant as you travel along. Pay attention to the detail and notice some of the small things that are of interest. Turn your head when you hear the call of a bird high above you in the sky, move to get the fullest possible view of the landscape around you from your vantage point, reach out and touch the water, rummage around in the drift of dried leaves and marvel at the sound they make.

Allow your mind to fill the screen with a richness of images and sights and relax as you let your body respond to them. When you are finished, remember to switch off the screen! Allow the curtains to draw back across it as the music comes up – you can come back again whenever you want.

Miscarriage

This is the spontaneous loss of a foetus during the pregnancy and can be very emotionally traumatic as well as physically demanding. The earlier in the pregnancy the miscarriage occurs the easier it can be to bear physically, the signs amounting to little more than a heavy period in the very early stages. Later in the pregnancy further treatment with herbs to cleanse the area after miscarriage, or even a surgical procedure (D & C), may be recommended.

The signs of miscarriage can range from blood loss to a sudden amount of clear discharge, accompanied by abdominal cramps. Consult your practitioner immediately you suspect any problem, and lie down.

The tremendous loss involved can often be overlooked and it is necessary to mourn and grieve for the loss of promise. There is often little formal structure or recognition for this type of grief, so it can be a very private affair. It is vital to take time off from regular routine and to attend to whatever feelings and emotions are surfacing. Professional counselling can be invaluable at this time.

One miscarriage does not necessarily mean that future pregnancies will not be successful and it is important to allay that fear at the earliest possible opportunity. The increased stress could have an impact on the future if it is not put to rest now.

Termination of pregnancy

Commonly known as abortion, this can be performed at any-time up to the twenty-eighth week, although in practice the limit is generally twenty-four weeks. There are many methods, depending upon the stage of the pregnancy, but some form of medical or surgical intervention is generally required. There are herbs that will work in the early stages to assist expulsion of the embryo, but these tend to have a terribly hard effect on the body. If you do not want the pregnancy to continue, some natural measures may be effective – stay very active, and spend time running and jumping. Swim using breast stroke leg kicks and focus your intention on what you are doing. If the pregnancy is not meant, it may just let go easily. (There is no reason to worry about swimming or being generally active if you want the pregnancy to continue. Here we are working with manifesting desire, and translating our wishes into physical reality.)

On an emotional level, this can be a very difficult procedure to decide upon, and there is often little support available. Feelings of grief and loss at the finality of the situation need to be acknowledged together with any resentment or guilt. This is also an opportunity to learn about forgiveness and experience further personal growth. We may need to forgive ourselves for choosing this event, or for the way we have behaved, or to forgive others for their role in it. If we believe in our own basic goodness or in the existence of the Creator, or any power greater than ourselves, then this may be an event that we can surrender to. Perhaps we can come to accept that for some reason this was necessary for us to experience, and that we have made the right choice.

Recovery

After any unsatisfactory outcome of pregnancy, whether through miscarriage, abortion or still birth, the body will respond well to any support and assistance. Treat with much love and care, just as when recovering from any other crisis. Aromatherapy massage with oils such as Rose, Geranium, Ylang-ylang and Sandalwood will help support the system and the emotions. These essential oils can also be added, two drops at a time, to bath water for the treat of a long soak at the end of the day. Attending to your feelings, although painful, is often the best way to recover. Giving yourself time on your own to work things through, and time in nature to get back in touch with your own cycles, are the two best gifts at this time.

Creative endeavours of any kind are excellent therapy, and often really personal or deep feelings that cannot even be spoken can come to the surface and be expressed through movement, singing, painting or creative writing.

Herbal remedies are most useful to strengthen and return tone to the system. Consider adding some sprigs of fresh rosemary to meals, and take one cup each day of lemon balm or weak Lady's mantle tea. Routinely add a strong tea made from a handful of thyme or calendula covered with boiling water and left to stand for thirty minutes to the bath water for their antiseptic qualities. Take ten drops of echinacea tincture in a little water each morning and evening for two months, to reinforce the immune system.

Ailments during pregnancy

As the foetus grows, the pressures on the woman's body increase. Any severe symptoms should prompt you to consult your practitioner straight away. Also, trust your instinct – if something doesn't feel right, pursue it until you get the satisfaction that you need.

Nausea

This may come and go during the pregnancy, but is often worst during the first few months, when the characteristic morning sickness can appear. The sense of taste is often heightened during pregnancy, so it is important to respond to that and change any remedies as you need to. Chewing a small piece of ginger root may be perfect at one point, then you may need to change to taking a cup of ginger tea or a glass of ginger beer. Other remedies to consider include weak lemon balm and lemon verbena teas, cinnamon sticks, and crystallised ginger.

Some women find relief from slowly eating a plain dry biscuit, or taking a piece of refreshing fruit. It is worth experimenting to find your own solutions by trusting your body and your taste buds.

Indigestion

This may get worse as the foetus grows bigger and presses up against the stomach. Eat smaller, more frequent meals, and consider substituting freshly extracted vegetable juices for meals on occasion. You may notice that some foods aggravate the indigestion, including fatty, fried and hot and spicy foods, and fizzy drinks. Gain immediate relief by chewing a few fennel seeds after eating, or adding a pinch of ground coriander to your meal.

Always remain upright for at least twenty minutes after eating, and do not lie down or go to sleep for at least one hour after a large meal.

Constipation

It is important to ensure regular bowel movements, so keep fluid and fibre intake high. Drink twice as much water as you think you need and concentrate on foods which provide natural fibre such as fresh fruits and vegetables, wholegrains, nuts and seeds. Walking is an excellent exercise to help move digestion along and stimulate bowel movements. Now more than ever it is important not to strain when you go to the toilet, and introducing your body to regular habits will be more effective in the long term. Start your day by slowly sipping a warm drink, and then sitting on the toilet for a few minutes. This will often be enough for your body to get the message and if you continue this routine a bowel movement should ensue.

Varicose veins

These large, uncomfortable veins which often lie just below the skin surface most often appear in the legs. Spend some time each day with your legs raised above the level of your heart – just prop them up on some cushions while taking your daily nap, or when relaxing in the evening.

Bathe the affected area at least three times each day with a wash made from calendula and witch hazel. Steep a handful of calendula flowers in a cup full of distilled witch hazel and leave to stand for about one hour. Strain the liquid into a bowl or bottle to keep in the fridge, and discard the flowers.

If discomfort is severe, squeeze fresh organic lemon juice directly onto the area, or cover with a cold arnica compress. Mix one teaspoon (5ml) of arnica tincture into about ½ pint

(290ml) of cold water, and add a small tray of ice cubes. Soak a clean cotton tea towel or other piece of fabric in the liquid, wring out so that it is not dripping, and apply.

Piles

These can worsen as pregnancy progresses and the pelvis tends to become more congested. Aim to avoid episodes of constipation by keeping the diet rich and varied, and drinking lots of water. Take lots of exercise, and do not spend too much time sitting in one position.

Apply comfrey leaves as a poultice to soothe and heal the area, or use a cold compress of calendula or Lady's mantle. Make up either of these as a cupful of very strong tea, then pour into a bowl or dish. Allow to cool and add a few ice-cubes to really chill the liquid. Soak a small pad of cotton wool in the liquid, lightly wring out, and apply, holding in place until all coolness is gone. Repeat with a fresh piece of cotton wool, until half the liquid is gone. Refrigerate the rest, and repeat later in the day.

If bowel movements are very painful, anaesthetise the area first by applying an ice-cube that is actually frozen distilled witch hazel or aloe vera, and keep another one to hand for immediately afterwards. You may also apply Swedish Bitters two or three times each day.

Backache

Your back is your support throughout pregnancy, and yet it has a conflicting job to do. It is affected by both the weight of growing pregnancy and the signals from hormones that are encouraging all the ligaments that hold it together to stretch and become more flexible.

Assist your back by moving correctly, avoiding any heavy lifting wherever possible, and learning what it needs. Keep your shoulders facing the same way as your hips, that is, avoid twisting movements, and keep your whole spine in the same plane. Wearing flat shoes will reduce pressure on the lower back, as will getting proper support when sitting. Experiment with cushions to get a comfortable position that offers good support to the lower back. Always support your knees with pillows when lying down on your back, and place a pillow between your knees when lying on your side to ease any tension in the lower back and hip.

Learning to bend from your knees rather than using your back and moving from the waist will also help. If you do lift anything heavy, keep the weight as close to you as you possibly can, and avoid any twisting movements. Massage your lower back regularly with St John's Wort oil, or have someone do it for you, or use an aromatherapy oil such as Geranium, Sandalwood or Chamomile diluted in a little carrier oil. Keep your back warm and add a little fresh ginger root and cinnamon to your diet to warm yourself up from inside.

Backache can be a way of alerting us to fears that we may have about the birth, or the outcome of the pregnancy, or whatever other things may be of concern. Or it may be a sign that you are feeling a lack of support, or have money worries. It is worth considering whether this plays a part in your backache, and what you can do to address it. If pain persists, consult an osteopath for a professional assessment.

Luciana, a vibrant thirty-year-old Italian woman, arrived at my practice when she was four months pregnant and experiencing terrible back pain in her upper back. She was the mother of a two-year-old, and was unable to lift him anymore because it hurt too much.

After some cranial treatment, I suggested a cold pack, and gave

---

her exercises to do as soon as she was able to move freely again. She was to apply the pack for three minutes, and then replace it with a warm compress to which she had added five drops of Rescue Remedy, the Bach flower remedy that is so good for treating any kind of trauma. She was to repeat this every two hours for the next two days, and it worked sufficiently well for her to be almost completely out of pain by the end of that time.

It was more important than anything that Luciana learn how to lift correctly in order to avoid damaging her back further, and still care for her toddler and the baby that was on the way. I repeated many times how she needed to keep her back straight, hold her child close to her if she was going to lift, and never twist while she was holding him. She made it into a little song in her own language which sounded wonderfully pretty, and she used to sing it to her son to soothe him, and to remind herself.

Her back pain disappeared after the second treatment, and she continued pain-free throughout the course of her pregnancy. She gave birth to an 8lb baby girl named Florence, and sings the same song to her.

Resources
Mamatoto The Body Shop, Virago
Natural Pregnancy Janet Balaskas, Penguin
Your Natural Pregnancy Anne Charlish, Boxtree
British Pregnancy Advisory Service 7 Belgrave Road, London SW1V 1QB. 0171 828 2484

Brooke Advisory Clinic 233 Tottenham Court Road, London W1P 9AE. 0171 580 2991

Miscarriage Association C/o Clayton Hospital, Northgate, Wakefield, West Yorkshire WF1 3JS. 01924 200709

BIRTH

Nothing else in life can ever really prepare you for this experience. After the long wait of pregnancy, birth can be a welcome relief. The signs are unmistakable – beginning with often subtle symptoms of increasing restlessness that can lead to some rather frantic nest-readying. Physically, practice contractions will have already begun a few weeks before the birth, vaginal discharge and pelvic pressure will both increase, and spurts of extra energy are often available.

Pre-natal classes will have given you information about what is likely to happen, and it is a good idea to have a labour plan and have a bag packed and a route worked out, know who is coming with you, what they need to bring, and so on.

This is it, then, the moment you will have waited certainly nine months for. Once the waters have broken and contractions have begun, you are likely to be too involved in the process to organise herbs, aromatherapy oils, etc. These can all be a very helpful adjunct to labour, and it is worth ensuring that whoever will be present to support you at the time of birth knows your wishes in relation to the way you wish to proceed. This is especially so when it comes to pain relief. There are many methods open to you – from the Lamaze-type breathing-based exercises which aim to focus your mind on something other than the pain, to pharmaceuticals and self-healing techniques of going right in to the centre of the pain and acting from there.

It is important to trust your own instinct as much as

possible. If you feel the urge to move around, follow it. There must be almost as many ways and positions in which to give birth as there are cultures. On this planet, women give birth squatting, lying in hammocks, kneeling, sitting over bowls of warm water, standing up, crouching down, and on all fours, as well as lying on their backs. Babies are born on dry land and in water, and are caught by midwives, friends, grandmothers, fathers, older sisters and doctors. Births are attended by shamans, families, friends, 'birthing sisters', strangers, only other women, or a partner. In some areas women are encouraged to scream and shout out our pain; elsewhere we are taught to save the energy and use it to push the baby out.

Births happen under the moon, in special birthing places, or hospitals, under trees, in steam baths, and near streams. Birthing women will be given silence, to honour their process, or listen to special music to help them centre themselves, have their bodies rubbed, massaged, oiled and steamed, depending on where in the world they are having their baby. In this essentially natural experience, all that is common about it is that it happens.

Managing Change

Giving birth is a momentous thing to do. Physically it will change you for ever, and psychologically and emotionally the effects will be long term too. It is important to prepare for this event. It is amazing how many women don't, and then the job of being a mother comes almost as a shock to them.

The nine or so months of the pregnancy should be one of the longest preparation periods for anything, but inevitably there are so many other concerns to be addressed and plans to be made that individual personal adjustment often doesn't get a look in.

As the time for birth approaches, it is more important than ever to leave aside practical and worldly concerns, and contact the other part of the self that needs to be honoured. Some people call that your inner child, or your body self, but the name doesn't matter at all. We can all identify that small part of us that seeks reassurance at this time, and that may have questions that need answering or concerns that need to be addressed before it can give of its riches.

Take some time to be on your own and talk to this part of yourself. You may find this easy to do out loud, or have a silent talk in the quietness of your mind or your heart. A good way to begin this dialogue is with two pens and some paper. Start by writing at the top of the paper whatever it is that you would like to say to this quiet aspect of yourself, perhaps asking it a question, or allaying an anxiety, or simply that you would like to talk. Then put down the pen, and with your other hand, the one you think you can't write with, pick up the other pen, and see what happens.

This is a wonderfully effective way of bypassing intervention from our thinking, rational selves into our emotional reality, and I have never known it to fail. Sometimes real written conversations are begun, or a small diagram or drawing that conveys real meaning will be drawn. It can appear to be almost magical, and is a very special way to instigate communication. Whatever your type of conversation, it is bound to be one of very real value, and if you are in any doubt, you may ask at the end of your talk whether there is any special gift or treasure that is now yours.

Our right brain, the side that thinks rationally and logically, governs the pattern of our understanding, and is all too ready to hear the voice of our intuitive, sensitive left side – it just takes a little help to begin the dialogue. This is a technique that is used by creative artists to unblock any potential flow or ideas, and can also be used to access our inner child, the subconscious or different aspects of ourself.

Another excellent dialogue to begin, if you have not already, is with your soon-to-be-born child. It is a very good idea to describe the process of the birth, and to reassure them, and yourself, that the outcome will be one of amazing joy and wonder, and that they will be most welcome.

Your Body Now

Giving birth can mark a turning point in our attitude towards our bodies, and often women are much more relaxed and freer after the experience. All the internal change, and the physical work of carrying the baby to this point will also have an effect on the body. Stretch marks are an obvious sign, although regular massage during pregnancy can help alleviate this; also the nipples are likely to remain darker, the lips of the vulva will be fuller, and the darkened line of hair that appears down the centre of the pelvis may remain. These can be seen as badges of honour that mark a woman's transition to motherhood.

The events of birth can be strong, but altogether positive, and there are many natural measures that can support and assist this essentially natural process. Many women respond well to being massaged, especially over the lower back and abdomen. This can be begun before labour starts, and may be appreciated right up until the final stages. Make a mixture of Clary Sage, Geranium, Rose and Ylang-ylang essential oils in a base of coconut, sesame or olive oil. All of these will have an affinity with the birthing process and will work on the uterus, or you may have a favourite which you prefer above the others.

Encourage your birth supporters to use a firm circular rubbing massage on your low back, and settle your energy there. Cover your abdomen with lighter, soothing strokes.

Use a simple hot compress (a towel dipped in hot water and wrung out) to soothe the whole abdomen by draping it over the bump, and replacing as soon as it cools. Make a strong infusion of chamomile or calendula, and soak a cotton cloth in this. Apply this warm compress to the top of the pubic bone, and leave in place till cool. This will bring relaxation and some relief from pain.

The atmosphere of the birthplace can help concentrate the energy and assist a smooth birth. Consider whether you feel more relaxed in subdued lighting, or prefer bright lights. Would you like the scents of burning cinnamon or dried lavender to cool you, or do you feel more reassured by antiseptic?

Do you need silence in order to connect with your inner self and really be with the process, or would you prefer music, or the sound of other women singing, or are you unconcerned? Consider all of these, and discuss them with a good midwife, or your birthing supporters. All of these factors can assist the mother enormously, impacting upon the feelings involved in giving birth. The process of giving birth is such a primitive one, that can seem to take over our bodies, and planning as much of the event as possible can also help us regain some element of control.

Of the many physical measures to help after the birth, pelvic floor exercises are the most essential.

PELVIC FLOOR EXERCISES

Strengthening the web of muscles that acts as a sling around the whole genital area will prove useful in many respects. It is essential to return tone to this whole region after childbirth, and this type of exercise can also help improve sexual satisfaction and bladder control. One of the easiest ways to identify the pelvic floor muscles is whilst urinating. Next time you are sitting on the toilet, endeavour to stop yourself in midflow. This is the exact movement that you need to make when you are not urinating to strengthen these muscles. Only do it to stop yourself actually peeing the one time; after you have identified these muscles you can do this exercise everywhere, and at just about any time. Begin by tightening them two or three times in a row and holding for a few seconds each time. Do this three times a day. Soon you will find that it becomes easy and that is the stage to increase the quantity and frequency of the exercise.

Now you can also exercise the muscles that would have you 'lift' or tighten your vagina, and, separately, your anus. Once established, you will be able to discern the smaller groupings of muscles and will be able to flex them at will.

What to Eat Now

In preparation for the birth many women find that their appetite changes significantly. It is quite common to lose a few pounds in weight in the days just before the birth, and there is no cause for concern if you have no interest in food. Sip a warm ginger drink at mealtimes to see if it will stimulate your appetite. Take a little finger-nail sized piece of fresh ginger root and cover with boiling water. Drink as soon as it is cool enough.

There are many herbs and plants that can be taken to prepare the pelvis for birth, and these can be started a few weeks before the birth is due. Take a little nutmeg, clove and cinnamon in meals for the last few weeks of the pregnancy; they will warm and prepare the abdomen for delivery.

Take a weak tea of raspberry leaf or motherwort every day for the last three weeks or so of the pregnancy to keep the pelvis elastic and relaxed. If feeling tired and weary, take some borage tea every day, or add chopped fresh leaves and flowers to salad meals and sandwiches. Sage is another useful addition to the diet, and fresh leaves can be added to a range of meals to act as a tonic in the final week or so.

If you intend to breastfeed, a number of foods will help to enrich your supply of milk. Adequate calcium is essential; help reinforce this in your diet by adding nettles, borage flowers and chamomile to your salads and other meals. Sesame seeds, kelp and other sea vegetables are also good sources. Onions and leeks will enrich your milk and lend it their antiseptic qualities.

Staying Well

- There are many natural measures and remedies that can support and assist the mother during birthing. Throughout the birth you can take weak herbal teas. When these are no longer tolerated, because of the volume of liquid, take them a few drops at a time from a dropper bottle, and place them under the tongue for instant absorption. Essential oils can be added for a foot or hand bath, and to massage oil for application to the lower back and anywhere else you would like.
- Take some fresh leaves of feverfew and sage and crush them under your nose to begin to strengthen and regulate contractions. Reinforce this by taking a cup of feverfew, sage or raspberry leaf tea. Regularly open and stretch the

mouth and jaw to release the uterine muscles. Lavender, chamomile and motherwort will increase relaxation and have a pain-relieving effect. Take these as a tea, or crush the fresh flowers of lavender under your nose, or dab the essential oil on the pillow, and massage some into the pulse points using a carrier oil.

- If contractions are over-strong make a warm raspberry leaf compress and apply to over the pubic bone, replacing as soon as it cools. Also consider massaging the lower back and legs with a mix of essential oils diluted in a carrier oil. Clary Sage, Rose, Ylang-ylang and Geranium are good choices, as are Olibanum, Chamomile and Rosemary. Crush fresh rosemary under the nose if losing awareness, and do so just before the moment of birth to assist the mind to clear and register the moment. Thyme has traditionally been associated with birthing rooms, and this powerful antiseptic herb can be crushed, or burned as an essential oil.

Managing stress

Arranging for the labour to be the way that you want it is just one of the potentially stressful situations that birthing can involve. It is so important to the success of the whole process that you feel empowered and satisfied at being able to make your nest just the way that you want it. Ultimately, though, there comes a time when you need to give it away, or hand over to the process itself, and trust that all will be well. This act of surrender is so important, and can seem very difficult when you are endeavouring to ensure the safety of your new-born for perhaps the first time. Nature helps, as always, if we trust it.

The pain of labour is perhaps another of nature's gifts. It

is certainly a definite way of grabbing our attention and ensuring that it is focused on the matter in hand. We can use this to great benefit if we can, once the time is due, focus inwardly and continue to concentrate on the birth process, rather than being moved by the fear and busy-ness of the situation. Whenever change is possible, there is also the possibility of fear – of the unknown, of so physical and primal an event, of failure, of pain, or whatever. Concentrating on the process itself, and what is required of you, will strengthen you and remind you of the love that is also a part of every element of creation.

Find a way to get in touch with the still centre within you that is ever-present, and constant in the face of all life's changes. This is a very strong place from which to give birth, or indeed to meet any challenge or trial. Sometimes the pain can act as a guide to finding that quiet place within. Gentle music may guide you there, or you may have experienced some form of meditation that will remind you of your way. Often all it takes is for you to relax, take a breath, and know that it is there. This place is absolutely and inviolably yours, it is a calm oasis in which to rest and rejuvenate, a well-spring of peaceful energy and a safe place to be. This is a good place to act from, and a place that allows you to make good decisions about how to proceed and what choices to make.

Often women have very strong feelings about the position they want to be in, or what they need to do to make their birth work for them. It is all too easy to be talked out of this by well-meaning professionals and others. It is essential that you listen to your body at this key time, and if you feel or intuit that something is good, then trust to it. It is a voice that comes from the deepest level of your experience, and it is sure to be good advice. The end result is likely to be a birth experience that is enhanced and enriched by your rooted sense of self.

Healing the perineum

Regular applications of cream throughout the pregnancy should have helped to soften this area and allow it to stretch enough for the baby to be delivered. If this has not been possible and the area has a tear, or has been cut (an episiotomy), speedy healing is essential. Bathe the whole area as frequently as you can with warm water, squeezing a sponge over the skin without actually touching it to minimise discomfort. Add a handful of sea salt to the water, or a strong tea made from St John's Wort.

Take homoeopathic arnica tablets for three days, and apply a warm comfrey poultice made from fresh root or leaves directly to the perineum for comfort and its speed of healing.

Post-natal depression

This is known as a reactive depression, or one that is occurring in response to all the enormous physical and emotional changes that occur around birth. Counselling and talking with people does help, and it is a first step towards treatment and recovery. Specialised care and advice is essential to ensure your return to total health, and a full nutritional assessment will benefit you enormously.

In the meantime, take one glass of pomegranate juice daily, and introduce time for yourself, finding someone else to care for the needs of your baby for just a little while each day. Even fifteen minutes can help. Dr Bach's Flower Remedies can be especially helpful, and if you are breastfeeding or do not wish to take them because of the alcohol involved, you can rub them into the pulse points of your neck, wrists, and behind your knees. Take or apply about five times a day. There is a specific range that can help with this type of depression, although you may feel drawn to any of the other remedies. Choose from Elm, Crab Apple, Larch, Sweet Chestnut, Star of Bethlehem, Willow, Oak and Pine.

Aromatherapy baths, foot soaks and massages can all make a tremendous difference; choose Sandalwood, Rose, Geranium, Howood and Thyme or Ginger. If you cannot have a massage, do it yourself, choosing parts of your body to work on at any one time. Foot and abdominal massages are amongst the easiest to do yourself, and the most rewarding.

Sore nipples

Apply small amounts of ghee to each nipple, reapplying as soon as it dries. You need not worry about baby sucking a little of this, it will cause no problem. If the soreness is bad, crush a handful of violet leaves and mix into a thick paste with a little warm water. Add a little runny honey, just enough to make it workable, and apply to each nipple. Cover with a piece of cotton fabric and put on a loose bra to hold the poultice in place. Keep on overnight or for as many hours as possible. Once removed, rinse each breast with warm water to which has been added two drops of rosewater. This can be repeated every night for a week, although good results should be seen after just one or two applications.

When a baby dies

The death of a baby is always a devastating event, whenever it occurs. It is vitally important that you talk about your feelings, and it may be appropriate to find a Bereavement Counsellor to support you in this. The feelings evoked are essentially personal, as with all grief, but they all need to be shared or aired. Stifling them and bottling them up is not a wise move in this situation – the tears need to flow, and there is great healing in their salty water.

It is good to feel the warmth of other human contact to remind us of the continuity of life, and massage from a caring professional or a loving friend is an invaluable aid throughout all the stages of mourning and recovery. Add a few drops of Rescue Remedy to the massage oil, and possibly some essential oils – Sandalwood is nice and supportive and helps with the fear of loss; Olibanum is useful to resolve emotional pain; Geranium is gently uplifting and can ease the sorrow. Trust your senses, and allow yourself to be drawn to any oil.

Keep yourself safe and warm, especially round the kidney and pelvis, and sit with a hot water bottle on your back to help you deal with the shock. Keep your feet warm, and consider taking hot foot baths with a handful of salt added to draw your energy down and back into your body. Work in whatever way you can on forgiveness.

Resources
See Pregnancy (p.169)

BABYCARE

There is a wealth of safe and effective natural solutions to all sorts of health concerns that face babies and young children. It makes good sense to begin treating infants with simple, natural measures and remedies because used properly they have no side effects, and will not set up any toxic effects. The straightforward natural remedies work by reinforcing the body's own healing efforts, and show effects remarkably quickly, mainly because babies' systems are still relatively pure.

It is a good idea to contact a Natural Healthcare Practitioner, who will be able to work with you to maintain and support your child's health. If someone can be found before or during your pregnancy, then so much the better. This is a particularly useful step if using natural measures is new for you, or if this is the first child you will be keeping healthy in this way. The support and encouragement of a practitioner will help allay any anxiety as well as providing professional support and assistance, and the vital job of ensuring correct diagnosis. Babies and children are not able to list their symptoms, or explain when any difficulty arose, so it is doubly important to make sure that any obvious concern is properly investigated.

Therapies to Consider

Cranio-sacral therapy and cranial osteopathy are techniques carried out by qualified practitioners. This type of treatment can be useful for all manner of baby and child complaints that prove stubborn or do not respond well to other forms of treatment. It can also be used for the mother to help her recover from the effects of pregnancy and labour. They seek to balance the baby's body after the traumas of birth. This is especially relevant if any form of intervention, such as forceps, was used during the delivery.

Jacky brought her three-month-old baby Jake to see me for some cranial work to help him get over a difficult, assisted birth. His head was still looking a little sore, and he was very grumpy, didn't seem to be particularly flexible in any of his joints, and was a poor eater. Jacky had begun trying to give him a bottle in between breast-feeds, fearing that her milk might not be good enough.

I treated Jake with some gentle cranial work to improve his sucking reflex and release any restrictions that I felt resulted from the birth. I encouraged Jacky to persevere with the breastfeeding, and to exclude wheat from her diet in case this might be irritating the baby. She was also to drink a cup of fennel tea each day to relax them both.

After the first treatment, Jake was particularly grumpy for a few days, but he was sleeping much better and managed to feed a bit more hungrily. By the end of the month, with two further treatments, and the dietary changes, Jake was feeding well and putting on weight. He was sleeping well and his body was slowly loosening up. His humour was also showing some slow improvement.

I continued to see them both once a month until we had identified a few foods that Jacky needed to avoid. His general outlook was very good, although he still had a tendency towards stiffness in the damp weather, and was never particularly good humoured. They left with a prescription for a regular baby massage, so that he and his mother could bond, and for careful attention to routine. A follow-up visit confirmed that, at one year old, Jake was thriving, and his mother felt quite happy with his progress and with their relationship.

Herbs too may be used to great effect with babies and children. External applications such as baths, poultices and packs are well received and safe to administer. Otherwise, single herbs may be given as very weak teas or indirectly through the mother's milk. It is worth remembering that whatever the mother is ingesting during breast-feeding, the baby is also ingesting. (Many cases of colic can be eliminated by the breast-feeding mother's avoidance of cows' dairy products.)

Baby massage

Babies respond terrifically to touch, and massage is a wonderful way for parent and baby to bond. Spending time in a warm environment, without the hindrance of clothes, and being gently and soothingly stroked by a loving mother has to be pretty close to bliss for a baby. It is a wonderfully healing experience for all involved, and once learned can be established as part of the daily or weekly routine.

The key to good baby massage is for the adult to remain relaxed, and convey only happiness to the baby in their hands. There is no point in becoming anxious about performing a stroke correctly, or including all the right techniques.

The essence of the massage is the bonding and pleasuring that occurs. Babies love to be touched, and respond wonderfully to being carefully and lovingly massaged. This is a perfect way to spend quality time together.

Start by getting comfortable. This can be sitting with a cushion on the floor, supported with pillows on the bed, or even at the kitchen table. You will need a towel to lie the baby on, and this can be draped over a large pillow, changing mat, or other soft surface. Massage can be done with just your hands (and this is best for babies up to one month old) or using a little gently warmed oil such as sesame or almond, to which is added a few drops of rose water. Never drop oil onto the baby's skin – use it to lubricate your hands, and then apply it. (Essential oils are not recommended for baby massage.)

Begin by using two types of touch – one long gentle stroke, and one small circular movement. Use the long stroke on all the long bones, i.e. down the arms and legs, and down the body; and make small circles around all the joints, e.g. shoulders, elbows and wrists.

With the baby lying on its back, you can start by covering the whole body with both hands stroking together, or one after the other, working down from the neck to the bottom of the feet. Use slow, gentle movements, and massage as much of the baby as you can, remembering fingers and toes, and spending a little extra time around the umbilicus. Do not use any pressure here, or on any other area – the strokes need to be light, continuous and rhythmic. The whole experience can be deeply relaxing or gently invigorating, depending on the speed you use. As a rule, slower is better.

If the baby is happy lying on its tummy, you can massage all of the back of the body in much the same way as you did the front. Otherwise, sit the baby up, either looking at you, or held closely with its back to you.

Lie the baby on its back again, and loosely cover its body.

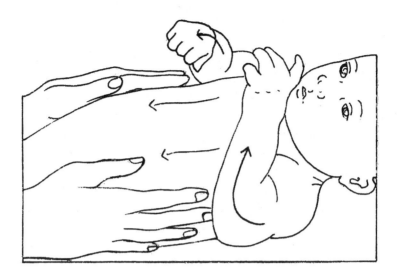

Using your fingertips, slowly stroke the face and head, down the neck and off the shoulders. Make these long, sweeping strokes that start near the nose and follow one after another sweeping the energy down and off the body. Gradually lighten the touch and reduce the speed of every stroke until you are barely touching the skin.

Finish the massage by making many strokes down the length of the baby's body to the feet. Stop and hold each foot gently between your hands for a moment, then do the same with each of the baby's hands. Rest your hand gently on the umbilicus area, and hold it there for a few moments, then finish altogether with the reassurance of a hug.

This is a wonderful way to round off bathtime, once baby is dry, but can be done at any point during the day.

Some days a few minutes will be plenty of time, on other occasions this can take up to half an hour, and may lead directly into a feed, or a nap.

Once you feel confident, you can incorporate different things, like gently tapping the soles of the feet, the palms, and the cheekbones with the tips of your fingers to stimulate circulation. Lift the limbs as you use both hands to stroke them, and lower them gently when you reach the ends. Use both hands to sandwich and press together exquisitely gently, all down the baby's sides. Use a light pulling movement away from the body as you stroke down the limbs and along the back away from the spine. Be creative. You will soon discover what your baby likes, and what is most appropriate to different moods. If the massage has been light and playful and energising, then it may lead naturally into some exercise, or gentle bouncing up and down. Otherwise it may spontaneously become nap time.

You may like to massage the baby on your bare tummy, while you lie on your back, or between you and your partner. Consider doing it outdoors in warm weather, and let the baby have an air bath at the same time. If the situation is not conducive to nakedness, you can massage very well through layers of clothes, by making each stroke a little bigger or more generous, and using a very slightly increased pressure. Consider, too, singing while you do this, or playing some appropriate music.

Beverley brought her baby Kerry to see me when she was four months old. The baby was unsettled and cried often, she seemed crotchety and was rarely calm. This was Beverley's first child, and she was a very anxious mother. She was very concerned about doing everything right, and making sure that her daughter got the very best of everything.

I had worked with Beverley a few years before and knew her

basic health was very good, and that she would have passed on her strong constitution to her baby. As we reviewed their daily routine, it became clear that, although using her best endeavours, Beverley was rushing through feeding and immediately jiggling Kerry up and down in order to burp her. I suggested slowing down, and relaxing some more, making surer that feeds were quiet, still, precious times, and that afterwards she simply hold the baby upright and gently rub her back. We also scheduled some appointments for Beverley to come back on her own and have some bodywork to settle her after the labour.

I referred them to a local homoeopath who would be happy to work with and support both of them, helping Beverley feel more confident in her ability to look after the baby. Within a week of starting the settled feeding routine, Kerry was settling down nicely. The bodywork proved to be very good for her mother, and within three months they were both getting along very nicely.

What to Do About Feeding Baby

Feeding

If it is possible, breast-feeding is a wonderful, natural way to give your baby the best possible nutritional start in life. It is also the time when deep bonding occurs and mothers often speak of falling in love with their baby all over again when feeding in this way. The stimulation that your baby receives at the breast will help in the development of their co-ordination and their breathing. This is an opportunity for the baby to establish the roots of good self-esteem as it receives large doses of mother's love and good nourishment. Remember that everything that you eat your baby will also take in through your milk.

Marshmallow leaf tea is very high in calcium and can be drunk regularly to improve the quality of your milk. Include small amounts of fennel, cinnamon and anise in your diet to increase milk flow. Take fresh thyme, sage, rosemary, garlic and ginger for their anti-bacterial actions and to help maintain both your immune systems.

Weaning

Everybody seems to have different ideas about the best time and way to do this. The arrival of the baby's eye teeth, often around eighteen months old, is a good sign that their own digestive systems are ready to take on a new challenge, but time and other restrictions usually determine when to wean.

Whenever it occurs, it can be a difficult time for both mother and child, so take it slowly. Both will inevitably miss the intimate time they spent together while feeding, however ready they might be to move on. This is an opportunity to continue the idea that sharing mealtimes with good company is a positive, health-enhancing activity.

- Make a tea for yourself from fresh sage leaves (red sage if possible) and drink it cold up to three times a day to dry up your milk.

Bottle feeding

Breast milk is undeniably best whenever possible, but if this is not available, do not be tempted to substitute it with cows' milk. This is a major source of food allergies and digestive troubles, and is not meant for tiny babies. The latest research shows strong links between cows' milk fed to infants and digestive complaints such as irritable bowel syndrome and Crohn's Disease later in life. There is also a great deal of suspicion as to the level of purity of baby's milk formula.

Goats' milk is much more easily assimilated. Home-made soya milk is not enough in itself to feed your baby, but it can be mixed successfully with goats' or breast milk, and rice milk is another good substitute.

Feeding times can still be very intimate. Some women lay their baby on the skin of their tummy, or at the breast whilst feeding with a bottle. This skin contact is immensely important, and alongside the eye contact allows the bonding that needs to occur between mother and child.

Keeping Baby Well

- Most babies and infants will respond wonderfully well to routine. Establishing regular times for eating and sleeping will often be enough to soothe and lull a slightly fractious or unsettled child. It is important to allow babies to rest after eating. Let them be still and settled for at least five minutes after each feed, only burping or bouncing them before that if absolutely necessary.
- If sleeping is a problem, sticking to a regular timetable will help. Adding a tiny sprinkling of cinnamon or a single black cardamom seed to flavour warm milk before bedtime will also soothe and settle. An evening bath to which is added a light infusion of lime flowers or lemon balm will aid relaxation and promote sleep. A good hydrotherapy measure is to soak a pair of cotton socks in barely tepid water, wring out well and put on at bedtime.

This does not cause colds or chills, and will encourage sleep very quickly.

- Cooled, lightly sweetened fennel tea made with ½ a teaspoon (2.5ml) of dried fennel makes a good alternative to gripe-water. (Fennel is one of its major ingredients.) Use a light sprinkling of cornmeal or cornflour as an alternative to talcum powder to keep baby dry. This is gentler on the body and holds no risks if inadvertently inhaled.

- If wet nappies are causing discomfort, a surprisingly effective alternative to powdering is to oil all around the bottom and thighs. Use a mixture of sesame or olive oil to which is added a small amount of rosewater, and a teaspoon of St John's Wort oil. During very hot or cold weather, a teaspoon (5ml) of cider vinegar may be added to check excessive perspiration. Keeping the area oiled deters nappy rash and means that no wetness seeps into the skin. If a rash has already occurred, wash with a dilute infusion of thyme or chamomile.

If you have any real concern about the health of your baby, consult your practitioner right away.

Cradle cap and other skin conditions

Skin complaints in breast-feeding babies can often be strongly influenced by mother's diet. Eliminating cows' dairy products, and reducing the amount of wheat may well show an improvement in the baby's skin within three–five days. This is also an ideal way to dose with herbs. During the spring and summer, the mother can drink one cup each day of nettle tea to ease the baby's troubled skin. During autumn and winter, take one teaspoon (5ml) of ghee with each meal. This can also be applied to the baby's skin and it will soothe and cool any irritation.

Young children eating solids can take one cup of quarter-strength herb tea per day for up to one week. They should also seek to avoid cows' dairy and wheat products.

Washing the affected areas with a diluted infusion of mallow, meadowsweet, or peppermint will show effects almost immediately. Treat any dried scabs directly with regular applications of sesame oil to which has been added a drop of rosewater. In severe cases, add one drop of Ti-tree essential oil to the mix. Ensure this is well dispersed before applying, and take care not to allow any of the mixture near the eyes or mouth. This powerful antibacterial and antiseptic oil will soon shift the most stubborn difficulties.

Change the bathtime routine so that soap is no longer used and is replaced by an oatmeal bag. Make this by enclosing a handful of oatmeal in a soft, cotton or silk handkerchief that is tied together to make a soft pad. This will gently cleanse the skin at the same time as being very soothing. Each small bag may be used two or three times. Alternatively, use an Ayurvedic herbal soap that will not alter the skin's acidity.

Ensure that this is not a reaction to some sort of allergy – babies can exhibit sensitivities to any manner of things, from wool to perfume. Things to watch for include detergents, alcohol-based scents, and especially men's aftershave. Young children can be very mobile, and it is worth paying close attention to their environment to rule out any contact allergy to soil, paint materials, or other substance.

Digestive upsets

Babies and children will develop their own digestive routine, so it is important to respect each individual child's needs and rhythms. Some children (like adults) will have one bowel movement a day, others will have three. It is quite natural for a child to be more in touch with their body's nutritional needs, so cravings for particular foods should be honoured – within reason. Also, do not worry if the child occasionally has no hunger. Do not force them to eat. This is a natural part of the body's digestive cycle, and will normally be followed by a day or two of increased appetite.

A cup of dill or anise tea made with ¼ teaspoon (1ml) of the herb and steeped for thirty seconds can safely be taken by infants past one month old. This has a calming, soothing effect on digestion, and is often enough to return things to normal after just one dose. It can be taken, if needed and showing a good response, for up to one week. Babies will respond well to a pinch of cinnamon added to a little warm milk. Calcium has a wonderful soothing effect on the stomach, so consider a spoonful of tahini or grinding sesame seeds and making into a thin gruel for children.

For colic, boil one teaspoon (5ml) of caraway seeds or aniseed with milk and feed the drink to the child for immediate relief. Alternatively, give 1fl.oz (28ml) of weak chamomile tea before and after each feed. If breast-feeding, remove wheat and cows' products from the diet, and drink the above mixture as well as giving it to the baby. Also take a cup of almond milk once a day. Make this by soaking 1oz (30g) of freshly grated almonds in one pint (570ml) of water for twenty-four hours. Keep covered in the fridge, and strain off and drink the liquid, discarding the almonds. This will help maintain energy levels, as well as soothing the stomach and topping up calcium supplies.

A small fingernail-sized piece of peeled ginger root added to a cup of boiling water will stimulate appetite after a period of abstinence.

Constipation and diarrhoea

Light massage is a wonderful way to stimulate a bowel movement. It can be incorporated into a regular massage session, or become part of the changing or bathing routine. Looking down at the baby's tummy, trace very lightly with your fingertips up from the top of the right thigh, across the tummy at the level of the umbilicus and down the left side of the abdomen towards the pubis. Repeat this several times, maintaining a light, stimulating touch, then make several light circles around the whole pelvis region following the same direction, i.e. starting from the top of the baby's right leg. Finish by placing your hand on the baby's abdomen and resting it there for a few minutes, allowing the heat from your hand to be absorbed.

To keep bowel movements regular, ensure that adequate water is being drunk and consider adding ¼ teaspoon (1ml) of slippery elm powder to warm water or dilute apple juice, and giving once a day. This will also help settle diarrhoea. Older children can increase the dose to one teaspoon (5ml) twice a day. A little stewed figs can be taken regularly to achieve the same results (strained for babies).

Diarrhoea can often be settled by taking warmed liquorice root tea to which one grain of salt has been added, sweetened with a tiny amount of honey. Consult your practitioner if symptoms persist for more than twenty-four hours.

Bowel movements are a good indication of digestive and overall health, and will be bound to fluctuate during periods of growth, changes in season and as a response to changes in the diet. Any ongoing difficulty should prompt you to take professional advice.

Fevers

In all cases, it is important not to panic. Consult your practitioner if you are at all worried, if the fever is high, or lasts for more than a few hours.

Sponge-bathe the infant with a dilution of two tablespoons (28ml) of cider vinegar in 1 litre (35 fl.oz) of tepid water. This will help reduce the temperature and soothe the child. Do not give any food, but plenty of just warm, weak fennel tea to drink. Make this by infusing a teaspoon of fennel leaves or seeds in a mug of boiling water for thirty seconds. Add one grain of salt and two of sugar. In the winter months, or if the child has a cold sweat that leaves them shivery, give garlic and ginger tea instead. Make this by boiling a 1″ (2cm) piece of peeled ginger root and ½ a peeled clove of garlic in one pint (570ml) of water for three–five minutes. Dilute with up to a pint of boiling water, and add just a dab of honey. Drink in sips once warm.

After a fever, the body needs to recover slowly, and the diet should be light and supportive to reflect this. In the warmer months, give mixed vegetable and dilute fruit juices for the first twenty-four hours, then proceed to a normal diet. During winter give a clear vegetable or potassium broth for the first day.

Teething

Calendula granules, available from your chemist or health-food shop, are wonderfully effective, and instantly soothe troubled gums. In the very early stages, a little honey mixed with one grain of salt may be rubbed into the gums. Liquorice and violet root are occasional treats to chew on once teething progresses, and leaves of fresh lemon balm can be given regularly. Take combination R tissue salt if breast-feeding, or feed to the baby directly. (You may want to check with your practitioner before doing this, but this is quite safe to do.)

Resources

A Gift from Sebastian Anne Diamond, Boxtree

Association for Breast Feeding Mothers 26 Holmshaw Close, London SE26 4PH. 0181 778 4769

La Leche League for Great Britain BM Box 3424, London WC1N 3XX. 0171 242 1278

MENOPAUSE

This is the natural cessation of periods in response to hormonal changes. It most usually occurs between the ages of forty-five and fifty-five, but may happen at any stage in a woman's life. It marks the end of our ability to conceive, but nothing else stops - while oestrogen production moves to other sites in the body, femininity, sexual ability and our creative talents and sense of self all remain intact. This can also be brought on earlier through the surgical intervention of a hysterectomy.

The first noticeable sign of approaching the menopause is likely to be irregular periods and this may begin as early as the mid-thirties. Once no period has occurred for two years, the menopause is said to be completed. This is women's third great 'secret', after periods and pregnancy, and is probably the final hormonal mountain that we are likely to climb.

This is an opportunity to make a new beginning, in the middle of our adult lives. A time to pause and evaluate achievements, and to make plans for the future.

Up to 80 per cent of women experience some symptoms, although one in five say this time could pass unnoticed. Amongst the wide range of possible symptoms, the most common are mood swings, hot flushes, tiredness and a lack of confidence.

This is a time of great change internally. The pituitary gland in the brain is stopping signalling the ovaries to produce oestrogen, so periods become erratic, and we begin to notice other changes. Other glands in the body, most notably the adrenals, slowly start to take over and produce the hormones we need, although in much smaller amounts than we have been used to. The hormones produced by the adrenal gland are stored in fat cells where they are converted into oestrogen, so body size is important here.

All hormonal activity is affected by the hypothalamus, the area of the brain that the pituitary gland is attached to, and this is very sensitive for regulation of our temperature, circulation, digestion, water balance, sleep, weight, emotional response, and bone structure: all the other areas that can become affected during menopause. Recognising this intimate connection can make sense of our experience.

Managing Change

This time can be challenging emotionally and psychologically as well as physically. Many women feel that they begin to be invisible within society. In our culture, with its focus on youth and sexuality, women can see the ending of their fertile years as an event to mourn. Look deeper, though, and you will see that life out of the mainstream of these pressures becomes no less relevant.

In other cultures and in traditional societies, postmenopausal women really come into their own. Freed of the responsibility that fertility carries with it, they can share their time and their wisdom with younger women, and concentrate on their own pursuits. More time is often available in which to pursue leisure interests, spend time with the extended family and other important people, and either continue to further life aims or make a change in direction.

Many women feel themselves to be entering a new era,

crossing some form of threshold into another stage in their lives. This can bring with it a renewed self-confidence, and a greater personal freedom. By the time we reach the menopause, many of us have usually managed to debunk the myths of competitiveness, and have seen enough of life to feel more comfortable within ourselves. Freed from the potential pressures of the sexual arena, many women feel free to explore their own sexuality, assert their own timing and sense of self.

This is the perfect opportunity to spend some time reviewing our past history, and assessing the certainty of our present course. Plans for the future will be stronger and clearer if any unfinished business from the past is cleared now. This is a little like weeding. If you pull out any deadwood at this point, the growth that remains is sure and strong. Begin your personal weeding by making a personal history.

MAKING YOUR OWN HISTORY BOOK

This is an excellent way to clarify your position and retune your wants and desires. You are going to make a project of your life to date, and assess the directions, choices and themes that you have followed up to now. This will enable you to make some clearer decisions about the path you intend to follow from now on.

Begin by dedicating a notebook or a folder or a scrapbook for this project. It needs to be something you will feel comfortable working in, so choose whatever feels right for you. I suggest that you start by writing your own story – the story of your life, starting with your birth and continuing right on to today. Ideally this should include all the important moments in your life, from your first day at school to your first love, etc. Include highlights, and low points, and the general feeling or tone of different periods in your life. Include your work life and your home life, your social world and more personal details. Where you can, include your hopes and dreams, your aspirations and goals.

This is quite a considerable job, and many women find they like to develop or explore certain areas while they proceed. If you are artistically inclined you may like to illustrate your story, or include photographs or any other mementoes that will enhance the memories of a particular time.

You might consider coding your entries into different sections of experience, or different areas of your life, e.g. career, home, emotional; or teenage, leaving home, becoming a mother. Work with this in whatever way you feel moved to until you have the story to date.

Then you will need to write a section on where you are right now – physically, emotionally, and in the world. This is more about how you feel and where you are in the process of your life.

Be brave, and write honestly. Nobody need ever see this, or you may choose to use it as the basis for your autobiography! Write about your relationships with those closest to you, with your family, and friends, and with your body, and your connection with Nature and the Creator. Write about what is important to you – your dreams and desires, what you want to achieve and where you want to be. Write about your wishes, and the reality of your situation, and how you manage your life on a daily basis. Include everything that you want to, and that you feel is important.

When you are finished, you will have a beautiful, personal, unique record of your life to date. The process of preparing it will have taken you through a review of all the important experiences that you have lived. You may well have cried and been moved by some of your memories, and laughed and rediscovered some forgotten episodes in your life.

You will certainly have steeped yourself in your history, and should have a pretty clear picture of where you have been, where you are right now, and what needs to be done next. This might be moving on in a particular direction, settling some unfinished business, or developing or discarding some aspects of your life.

The project itself is a wonderful thing to keep, or can make a truly loving gift to a child. You might choose to commit it to the elements as a give-away, or have it encased in plastic and placed on show in your home alongside any other great creative works. The decision about this and the rest of your future is yours.

Your Body Now

The physical signs all point towards this being a time for rest and renewal. Your body is going through a great change, and it is important to keep your focus on your own nurturing. Find ways to be kind and supportive to yourself, and allow time for rest and stillness. Make sure that relaxation is high on your agenda, and reschedule your life wherever possible to allow more time for this on a regular basis. Reassess those things, activities and pursuits that you find relaxing, and make sure that you give yourself the time to enjoy them.

Balance this with twenty-minute sessions of weight-bearing exercise at least three times a week. This helps keep your body in shape and guards against osteoporosis. If you have never exercised in your life, now is the time to do it. Begin slowly, and work up to a commitment to regular exercise. Weight training, dancing, running, and aerobic-type classes are all good exercise, and walking is the perfect way to achieve good aerobic exercise and a full body workout. Walk with a friend or friends, choose places that you like and make sure this becomes an enjoyable part of your life, that way you will continue to do it.

AIR BATHS

Skin is a tremendously receptive, responsive organ, and regular stimulation is important for ongoing good health. Take a few minutes every day to take an air bath – make it part of your morning routine, and feel the benefits throughout the day.

Stand naked with some good clear space around you for air to circulate, or in warm weather stand near an open window. 'Bathe' yourself in the air, covering as much of your body as you can by moving your hands just above the surface of your skin, as though you were splashing your body with water. Pay particular attention to the soft places like the underside of your arms, the backs of your legs and the soles of your feet. Let yourself enjoy the slightly exciting physical sensations as the air caresses and cleanses all around you.

When you have covered your whole body, not forgetting your head, stand still for a few moments with your eyes closed and your arms outstretched. Simply enjoy the feeling of the air all around and all over you, and imagine your whole body breathing, letting the air move into you and out of you in a continuous cycle of movement.

What to Eat Now

The menopause brings with it many symptoms and a wide range of health concerns. Many of these can be directly attributed to the enormous change that the body is experiencing, yet some can also be the signs of general health imbalance that are coming to the surface at this time. These can often be overcome using our knowledge of the nourishing and curative values of foods.

Food is an instant and excellent way to support your body through this time of change, and ensure the best possible range of nutrients. Begin by including all the foods and herbs that are rich in oestrogen and oestrogen-like substances in your diet as regularly as possible. This can make an enormous difference to your feelings of well-being and will ease the transition away from ovarian production to adrenal work, and can be done easily by having an oat-based cereal for breakfast, and at least one main meal salad each day. Add a range of fresh herbs and flowers to the salad meal and experiment with soya for cooked dishes.

Oestrogen-rich foods to include regularly in your diet are:

- sprouted seeds
- whole grains in moderate amounts
- bananas
- oats
- soya in all its forms (tofu, mung, miso, etc.)
- alfalfa
- celery
- anise, fenugreek, sage, calendula, fennel, liquorice and ginseng.

Vitamin E also stimulates the production of oestrogen, and favourite sources include avocados, seaweeds, leafy vegetables, milk and milk products, nuts and seeds. Check your blood pressure before taking as a supplement, but if all is well then take up to 1,000IU a day as a crisis management dose, and reduce once your body has begun to rebalance itself. Vitamin B and zinc are also important and can be taken as part of a multivitamin and mineral formula.

Now more than any other time, minimise the disruptive effects of stimulants on your body, and avoid caffeine, too much neat sugar, and alcohol. If you smoke, stop.

The other main area of concern is to ensure sufficient calcium in the diet to protect against osteoporosis. Good sources of calcium include milk, green vegetables, nuts, seeds – especially sesame and all its products (halva, tahini, Gomasio, etc.), dried fruit, soya beans and bony fish. Parsley, dandelion leaves, nettles and kelp are also good sources.

Calcium needs other factors in order to work well in the body, notably magnesium, boron and vitamin D. Magnesium can be found in many fresh fruits and vegetables, as can boron. Vitamin D is found in sunlight so it is important to get out into the air and let our skin be touched by the light on a regular basis. It is also present in fortified foods such as margarines and in oily fish. It is a good idea to take an all-round vitamin and mineral supplement at this time, but especially one which contains calcium and magnesium, boron and vitamin D to enhance calcium effectiveness. Specially balanced formulas are available from nutritional suppliers.

Take a weak tea made from equal parts of hops and agrimony as a general tonic once a week. Drink in the early part of the day and finish before it becomes cool. If your skin is dry as a result of the drop in oestrogen levels, drink calendula or chamomile tea daily. Calendula is high in oestrogen, and chamomile also has anti-inflammatory and calming properties. Make all of these by soaking one teaspoon (5ml) of the herb or herbs in boiling water for about fifteen seconds before removing.

I first saw Margaret because of some digestive complaints. An attractive, well-groomed woman in her late thirties, she felt she was not digesting her food very well, and was concerned that she was losing weight. She seemed worried and quite distracted, not being interested in telling me about her health history, but keen on expressing her anxiety about the future.

She didn't want to be a shrivelled-up old prune before her time. Her skin was important to her. These and other concerns made it quite clear that she felt she was approaching the menopause. She had not had a period for two months, and was very concerned, but she did not want to go to her GP in case he told her that she was not suitable for HRT.

I asked if she had always been this jittery, or felt this much concern about her future. It emerged that this was quite a recent thing, and had all started a few months earlier. Margaret had been under considerable stress at work during the previous year, and I felt this was the most important fact in her case. I managed to convince her that it was worth learning some stress reduction techniques whatever the true diagnosis was, and that relaxation was important. She agreed to spend thirty minutes twice a day with some techniques, and also took a B-complex supplement, with manganese and calcium to soothe her nervousness and settle her. She changed her diet to include more oestrogen-rich foods, and promised to have regular mealtimes.

At the end of the first month she experienced mild cramping with the full moon, but no period arrived. She did, however, feel 'smoother, less anxious', and was persevering with the relaxation skills. By the end of the third month she had a pain-free period, and was feeling quite energetic and happier again. She had regained the weight she had lost prior to her first visit, and was again enjoying her food. Six months later she has regular periods, not unusual for a woman of her age, and we have scheduled an appointment for next year to discuss her preparations for the menopause in good time.

Staying Well

- A herbal moisturiser will prevent the skin from losing too much moisture, and protect against outside influences. These are easy to make and very pleasant to use. Apply twice daily, morning and evenings, for best results.

Mix together two tablespoons (28ml) each of glycerin, rose-water and marigold water. Whisk these together and store in a screw-top jar. To make marigold water place 1oz (30g) of marigold petals in a pan with two cups (450ml) of water. Simmer very gently for thirty minutes and then strain and add 1oz (30g) of fresh petals. Make the rosewater in a similar way, but store for three days before using to allow the more delicate flavour to fully infuse.

- Another, slightly heavier moisturiser can be made by melting one tablespoon (28ml) each of lanolin, honey, almond oil and white wax in a bain-marie. (Stand a bowl over a saucepan that has a small amount of boiling water in it. This way you benefit from the heat without any risk of burning the ingredients.) Remove from the heat and add two tablespoons (56ml) of a strong infusion of lime or violet leaves. Leave to cool slightly then whisk until thick and creamy and pot up. If you are allergic to lanolin, substitute extra honey.
- Every morning, take a short barefoot walk on a patch of clean grass. If it is wet with early-morning dew, so much the better. This is an age-old remedy that works on many different levels. It is a stunningly immediate way to reconnect with the elements of the natural world, and you will continue to feel the benefits throughout the day.

Managing stress

Stress can affect us at any age. When it is good it can challenge and motivate in a powerful way, but it is necessary to have spells of time that are stress-free in order to rest and revitalise. The physical changes of the menopause often occur around the same time as any mid-life crisis, so there may be both internal and external stresses to deal with. It can feel as though we are just coming to terms with life and career decisions, and then we need to deal with all this physical change as well.

This is the time simply to stop. Just take time out and do nothing. Not reassess, not find another solution, choose a new way, or analyse the situation, simply rest and relax and allow ourselves to be renewed and refreshed.

Spending time in Nature is a wonderful way to allow this renewal to happen. Taking gentle walks, or just sitting near a tree and enjoying the magic and wonder of the natural world is powerful healing. Make a point of doing this every day. It is as important to your nourishment and well-being as eating and sleeping.

COLOUR HEALING

Sit or lie in a comfortable position and take a few deep, relaxing breaths deep down into your belly. Choose a colour that you like from the cooler end of the spectrum, e.g. blue, lavender, lilac, purple, yellow, green, light pink or white.

Close your eyes and imagine that colour in a ball right in front of your eyes, a vivid pulsing ball of strong bright light that radiates gentle warmth and a good feeling. Do not mind if the colour changes or fluctuates, it will settle into the colour that you need.

Hold the ball of gleaming, coloured light in front of you, and watch as it oscillates and twinkles, shining ever brighter and brighter until it appears like a sun, almost dazzling in its brilliance. Be aware of the intensity of the light and how it radiates warmth and good feelings.

Feel the glow of the coloured light gently touch and warm you, letting you relax into the comfort of its brightness.

Now take one big, deep breath in, and with it however much of the sunlight as feels comfortable, taking it right inside you. Keep the light there, as you breathe out, and return to normal, relaxed breathing. Feel the warm glow deep within you pulsing slightly and radiating a gentle warmth like its twin outside your body. Now you have a sense of what it is like to be a planet that has two suns!

Stay relaxed, and experience the love and warmth that is both within you and without. Allow the warmth to glow and grow until you are completely filled and surrounded by the warm, healing light. Keep breathing and stay basking in the light for as long as feels comfortable.

This is an exercise that you can repeat daily. The intensity of the experience will develop as you become used to working in this way, and you will be able to remain longer, basking in the glory of the light.

Hot flushes

These and night sweats are quite common early symptoms. They tend to appear quite suddenly and last up to a couple of minutes each time. Wear only natural fibres, and dress in layers so that it is easy to remove one.

Stress, worry and nervousness will all make each attack worse, so develop a way of relaxing that works for you.

Avoid hot drinks and spicy foods, plus red meats, alcohol

and cheese. Chew a pinch of fennel seeds after each meal, and add cooling spices like coriander seed to occasional meals. Include cooling foods like cucumber and borage leaves, and begin your meal with a small salad or chilled soup. Place some liquid aloe vera in a perfume spray or mister bottle, and add two drops of Rose essential oil. Carry this with you if possible, and use to spray and cool the face, neck and other accessible areas.

If you do not have high blood pressure, take a vitamin E supplement of 400IU a day, rising to 800IU over at least six weeks.

Emotional changes

A range of difficulties from sudden mood changes to depression, irritability and anxiety can occur during the menopause. Sudden fears or worries can take on greater than usual importance. Taking regular exercise is invaluable for the sense of natural rhythm and the good feeling it promotes. In the absence of any other measure, this would be the treatment of choice.

Finding the energy to undertake a regular programme comes from a good, varied diet, and working with any emotional issues as they come up so that nothing is suppressed.

Seeing a counsellor is a good way to address any issues as they surface, but so too is talking with friends and family, and writing about your feelings. Just talk to anyone or anything that will listen. Get lots of support from those around you, and if possible talk to your mother and other family members to learn about their experiences of this time.

Have regular massage with uplifting essential oils like Geranium and Jasmine. Add a few drops to the bathwater along with Ylang-ylang and Olibanum to relieve the worries and rebalance your system.

Take a broad-spectrum B-vitamin supplement to help with depression. Vitamin E will help with headaches and nervousness.

Many women speak of a lack of confidence at this time, or an inability to cope. Knowing that you are doing the very best for yourself can help you to centre yourself and relax a little more about your image in the outside world. Review who you are, rather than who others might think you are. Your identity is not all about your ability to have children, and that is all that has changed. You are a wonderful, unique woman, with memories and experiences and knowledge that is different to every other living person on this planet right now. That is quite something to be proud of.

Keep moving, and concentrate on the images of mobility and change. Focus on the change that is occurring in your world rather than trying to get on with your life as normal. Become a changed woman, and walk the truth of your new life.

Tiredness

This is a common complaint, and this time really does take its toll on the body's energy reserves. Reorganise your schedule wherever possible to include extra time for rest and relaxation. Consider taking an afternoon nap, and always have a stroll outdoors when you can simply meander along and be at one with your thoughts and feelings. As far as possible introduce a regular schedule for bedtime, and get an extra hour or two before midnight.

Concentrate on the transition phases between events, and let these replenish you – mark the end of the working day with a stroll outdoors, finish the evening with some quiet time to rest and reflect on the day, and cultivate the quietness needed for restful sleep. Take a short break between different daytime activities to regroup and order your thoughts and focus on the next project.

Ensure your diet is top notch, concentrating on natural foods wherever possible rather than those that are chemically grown.

Debbie came to see me because she hoped I would have some advice for stemming her copious bleeding. She was forty-nine, and her periods seemed to be lasting for longer and longer, and getting heavier. She was feeling quite drained and exhausted, and very irritable. She had hoped that the menopause meant her periods would stop, not that they would become more profuse. Medical tests had confirmed that there was nothing sinister going on, and her busy GP had little time and no other suggestions for her.

She started taking a multivitamin and mineral supplement, and one cup of Lady's mantle tea every other day, along with lots of oats and mung beans in her diet. She also included a lot or iron-rich foods, and plenty of roughage and natural fibre from fresh fruit and vegetables to help clear the pelvis. She ate a convalescence-type diet with lots of warming foods, and soups, to comfort and strengthen her. After two weeks her next period began, but she said she was feeling stronger in herself, and found it less tiring.

She increased the strength of the multivitamin, and began taking regular long walks to keep the pelvis mobile and tone her whole body. She took a protein supplement, and began to listen more to her body's needs. Once she was feeling strong enough, we planned a series of two day-long fruit fasts, timed to coincide with ovulation, and during that time she also took a modified Sitz Bath each day.

She said she had never worked so hard with her health, and yet was truly enjoying the experience.

At the end of six months her bleeding was under control, and she reported feeling better than she had done since she was twenty. She has a massage or an aromatherapy treatment every month, and comes back to see me every six months. We are waiting to see what her body needs her to do next, and in the meantime she maintains an excellent standard of nutrition, walks regularly, and feels good in herself.

Sex

Little need change in our sexual lives as a result of the menopause. Some women feel that the relief from the need to use contraception to prevent pregnancy frees up an aspect of the experience for them. Changes in libido are common, and the rate of vaginal secretion may drop slightly. All measures that reinforce feelings of femininity and sensuality will work wonders, and massage of the whole body, or just the pelvis region is a wonderful and instant way to do this. Add two drops of Rose and Ylang-ylang essential oils to the mixture to stimulate desire and reawaken physical yearnings, or add your own favourite scent.

Address any feelings of loosing femininity, or lack of attractiveness that could be at the root of any difficulty. The range of Bach Flower Remedies are a powerful aid to restoring self-esteem and can be taken as directed or applied to the pulse points. If any seem especially relevant, a drop or two can also be added to massage oil, bathwater and to drinks.

Add garlic, rosemary and cinnamon to your diet to strengthen your sexual response, and consider taking five drops of myrrh tincture each day in a small glass of water. This is an age-old tonic for the whole reproductive system.

Coconut, sesame seeds, olive, almond and peach nut are all excellent oils to use externally to stimulate the body's own secretions. This is an opportunity to linger in the area of arousal and stimulation, because the body will respond, only it may take a little longer. Relax as much as you can and enjoy the experience. If the idea of sex or lovemaking is totally unappealing, and you have addressed any issues of intimacy with your partner, then consider talking to a counsellor or consult your practitioner. Every woman responds differently, and it is important to recognise your own needs as completely normal, even in such a sensitive area as this.

Osteoporosis

When there are problems with or a sudden fall in the body's oestrogen levels, a whole chain of reactions occurs. One of these is a tremendous impact on calcium levels, and on the density of the bones. This can cause problems making us feel more frail and vulnerable, and likely to break bones more easily. It also accounts for some of the postural changes we will experience. There is much we can do to guard against this, and the most powerful thing is to continue taking regular weight-bearing exercise. This can be as simple as walking, an excellent all-round exercise, but it needs to be regular and sustained.

- Take weight-bearing exercises daily, or at least three times a week. This can be as simple as walking, when you are carrying your own weight. This has a protective factor on the bones and is one of the most effective measures you can implement for overall health.
- Take extra care with your diet, ensuring good sources of

calcium, magnesium, and oestrogen-stimulating herbs and foods. Do not focus on dairy foods, but get calcium from a wide variety of different sources including sesame seeds.

- Be moderate in your diet with any foods that can interfere with calcium absorption, e.g. whole grains and bran, which contain a substance that can interfere with absorption, and also oxalic acid-containing fruits and vegetables which do the same thing, e.g. rhubarb, spinach, sorrel and tomatoes.

- Supplement with boron, calcium and magnesium, and vitamins B and E. These are all involved in ensuring and regulating adequate calcium absorption, and will top up any long-term dietary deficiency.

- Ensure regular outdoor contact and dietary sources of vitamin D. This too is essential to the maintenance of healthy bone.

- Upgrade your dental care, and ensure regular cleaning and check-ups. Teeth are often one of the first sites to show bony deterioration.

- Take one cup of Lady's mantle herb tea every week without fail. This is a wonderful herb for women at this time. Its common name describes the area of the body with which it has most affinity, the mantle referring to the pelvic region. Steep one teaspoon (5ml) of the dried herb in boiling water for thirty seconds and drink before it cools.

- If you do break a bone or suffer with spinal compression, apply comfrey compresses made from the leaves or root of the plant. Keep reapplying as often as you can. If you are in a cast, tuck some fresh leaves in to let their active properties be absorbed through the skin.

Resources

The Menopause Handbook Dr Sandra Cabot, Boxtree

Health Information Service 0800 66 55 44

National Osteoporosis Society PO Box 10, Radstock, Bath BA3 3YB. 01761 432472

GROWING OLDER

Increasing years present their own challenges and opportunities. Our attitude towards the whole ageing process will influence how well we feel physically and emotionally. Old age and ill health are not synonymous, and it is never too late to instigate good and enjoyable health measures.

As we age we may have to work a little harder to maintain energy levels and general fitness. Any extra effort pays dividends, and reinforces the body's best intentions for staying well. We may have more time now to devote to the quality of life and our own health and welfare. Increased fragility, loss of speed and suppleness can all be accommodated or adapted to. The very real benefits of a lifetime's experience, knowledge and wisdom outweigh the majority of minor physical restrictions. Good nutrition, regular exercise and outdoor contact and intellectual stimulation will maintain a positive level of well-being.

Age is not honoured in our society as it is in other more traditional ones. This cultural poverty is not based in fact and it is important to remember that when we recognise positive attributes within ourselves we become more able to dismiss any external prejudice.

It is often in later years that our thoughts reach beyond our worldly concerns to more spiritual matters. Questions about our purpose and the meaning of life, and what the future may hold, may all enter our minds. Finding the answers that are true for each one of us can be one of the most satisfying and rewarding activities that we have ever pursued.

Women tend to live longer than men, and as over sixty-fives we form the fastest growing group in the Western world. This opens up the possibility of great support and company from a wide community of other women, a necessity when we face the grief of losing friends and partners.

It is important to remain active on as many levels as possible. Obviously physical agility must be maintained, and any gentle exercises that increase suppleness can be included as part of a daily or weekly routine. Mental agility can be maintained by remaining interested – indeed, following your heart is good advice for every stage in life. This is the time when old dreams can be reawakened, and things we have always wanted to be able to do can be achieved. For many of us, this will be the first opportunity to do just what we want to do, or to have the time to devote to what we want. It is a wonderful opportunity to review our life and reconsider our plans for the future, but it is also the perfect time to instigate some action and begin projects that we may have been putting off for years. Action carries its own rewards, and just beginning something can have spin-offs in terms of keeping our energy moving, our attention captured and our motivation fuelled.

There are many physical treatments that can be seen as treats and that are really good for us in later years. Being able simply to receive the good energy and allow good feelings in the body from a range of therapies is tremendously good. Massage, reflexology, aromatherapy, zero balancing, and cranio-sacral therapy are all worth considering, along with saunas, steam baths, jacuzzis and float tank experiences. The emphasis can truly be on enjoying life and the richness of it all.

Managing Change

Freed from the sense of being driven to achieve profession-ally and sexually, many women can enjoy this as a time with-out pressing career and family commitments. Time is available for reflection and for more creative pursuits, and to fulfil a different kind of role in the world. As older women we can speak with our own authority, and teach others the value of wisdom and experience, alongside youth and learn-ing ability. From here we may also offer advice and assistance within our own extended family and the wider community.

It is not always an easy thing for us to speak out with knowing and confidence. This is especially true when it relates to personal matters such as our feelings and experiences. One of the challenges of this time of life is to find the ability to share what we know in the knowledge that it may be good for others to hear it so that they may learn from us.

Although women can be role models and mentors at every stage of life, it is later in life that we most often feel we have both the time and the experience to fulfil this position. Many women see this as a way of being able to 'give some-thing back' or to enable younger women to benefit from their experience and wisdom. Of course, many of us do not call it that, we simply help out, with families, in the work place, or with charities and voluntary groups.

It is good to remember that there are many younger women who could benefit from hearing about your achieve-ments and sharing your time. There is a wide range of venues for such good work, ranging from formal 'women in busi-ness' groups, to those in a special area of interest or expertise, like charity, or political work, dedicated social groups, and religious or spiritual groups. You may also consider that whatever you do, you have the opportunity to influence everyone that you meet, in every situation. When you are true to your own beliefs and 'walk your talk' then you can have a profound effect on every area of your life.

As we grow older and by necessity develop relationships that include an element of dependence, giving of our knowledge and experience can be a way to balance our need. It is other women who will tend to be the carers who will look after us in later years, and often family members. They can benefit enormously from the rich reserve of family knowledge that you can impart.

The following exercise is a powerful one which if performed every day can have an amazing effect upon the way you feel, reinforcing your sense of purpose and your unique position in this world.

THE BRIDGE

Stand with your feet a few feet apart, and raise your hands up and away from your body, so that you are making an 'x' shape with your body. Keep your neck and the rest of your back relaxed, and reach out slightly with your arms until you can feel a very gentle stretch. Move your legs apart slightly until you begin to feel your body become taut. Close your eyes and take a deep breath.

Keeping your eyes shut, begin to imagine the energy of the earth moving up gently through your body from the contact that you have on the soles of your feet. Feel it rise through your whole body and travel up your arms to your fingertips and beyond. Relax and, keeping your breathing steady, enjoy the feeling of grounding that the earth is giving you.

Now, without disturbing that gentle energy flow, imagine the energy of the heavens slowly descending through your body from the top of your head, and the tips of your outstretched fingers. Feel it fall easily through your whole body reaching all the way down to the ground where you stand. Relax, and keep your breathing steady. Feel the sense of inspiration and light that now fills your body, and enjoy your position as bridge between earthly and celestial energy.

Hold this position for as long as is comfortable, then open your eyes, and slowly lower your arms and bend your knees slightly to release your lower back. Take a few deep breaths and review your experience.

Pauline was a charming and quiet woman in her sixties. She first came to see me with a minor skin complaint which cleared up as soon as she began taking a multivitamin supplement and applying some vitamin E oil to the area. Her next visit was about some backache, which cleared up after one treatment. Then she made another appointment to tell me of some indigestion she was experiencing. We dealt with this very quickly by changing her diet so that she ate smaller meals, and ate more often during the day.

I wondered if she might be lonely, and the next time she called for an appointment we discussed the matter. I suggested that maybe she had been given this time on her own to deepen her relationship with her own self.

We talked about nothing else during that session and she said it was the first time she had ever spoken of those feelings with anyone because she didn't want to 'make a fuss'. Since her husband had died, her social life had dwindled and she lived alone, so sometimes didn't see anyone at all unless she made the effort to get out to the local shop.

We scheduled some reflexology treatments with a local therapist, so that she would still feel the touch of another person, and this can be a very chatty experience, too. We also discussed some other options, including getting involved in some charitable organisations who are always keen to have volunteer help. She seemed considerably brighter after having faced the problem.

When I next saw her, three months later, she was feeling a lot more confident. She had regular commitments on three days of every week, and admitted to actually enjoying time on her own now. Her health had improved, and she continued to take a multivitamin supplement, with extra vitamin C to provide additional energy when she felt she needed it.

Your Body Now

As we get older our bodies change from being more physically able and supple, and it is important to retain our ability to move around as well as we may. Gentle, regular exercise will keep most joints supple, and walking is a wonderful way to combine rhythmic exercise with being out in the open air and staying in contact with nature.

Often any frustration we may feel at being slower or less dextrous is made much less significant by the love and care that we have by now learned to have for our bodies and our own way of doing things. If not, then it's never too late to learn! Imagine what compassion you would have for a friend who was endeavouring to do all that they could to please you, despite their awkwardness or frailty. Extend this love and forgiveness to yourself, and you can experience a whole new way of living.

We will necessarily see some postural changes as the

bones of the spine lose some of their density, and the discs in between them no longer spring back into shape. Gravity also takes its toll, and some form of spinal curvature or stoop is almost inevitable. Regular, gentle exercise – even if it is something very, very simple like some fluid arm movements, will help retain mobility in this area, and reduce any risk of headaches, neck tension and other complaints.

Keeping physically fit is very necessary. Chi exercises are especially good.

Chi

Chi is the Chinese word for that vital energy or spirit that animates us. It is universally acknowledged: the Japanese call it Ki, it is Prana in Hindi, and is also called Manna. Through focusing on this energy we can reinforce our own vitality. It is important to recognise that this is a way of making contact with the universal energy that surrounds and supports us, and that is available to us whenever we accept an end to separation.

These warm-up exercises increase Chi or vitality. They can be done every day as a gentle exercise or to focus attention on your body's energy. If you enjoy the experience you may choose to investigate Qi Gong (or Chi Kung) classes, Ki work or T'ai Chi.

LOWER BODY

Begin by standing quite relaxed with your feet together pointing forwards. Bend your knees and rest your hands loosely on your thighs, just above each knee. Relax your neck and shoulders, and centre your gaze on a point about six foot (nearly 2m) in front of you on the floor.

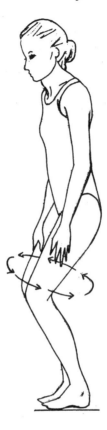

Keeping your knees together and your feet flat on the floor as much as possible, make twelve slow circles in an anti-clockwise direction with your knees. Take it nice and slow, and remember to keep breathing. Pause for a moment after completing the twelve circles, and take a deep, cleansing breath. Now make twelve circles in a clockwise direction, and finish with another deep, cleansing breath.

You may hear a few cracks and clicks as you go through the movement, and these are nothing to worry about, although you should stop immediately if you feel any pain.

Move straight into the next exercise.

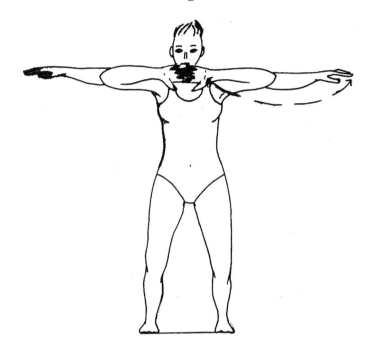

UPPER BODY

Stand quite relaxed with your feet flat on the floor about hip-width apart, and facing forward. Let your arms hang loosely by your side, and keep your neck and shoulders relaxed. 'Sit down' slightly by bending your knees out over your feet, and keep your bottom tucked in and your back straight.

Take a big breath in as you raise your hands to chest height, with your palms facing away from you. As you slowly breathe out, push your arms gently out in front of you as though you were starting a breast-stroke swimming movement. At the end of your exhalation pause for a second. Sweep your arms around and back towards your body as you inhale, completing the breast stroke. Repeat this twelve times, taking each breath nice and slow, and allowing the movement to glide. Imagine it is as fluid as the water you would normally be moving through. Finish by allowing your hands to fall back gently to your sides. Take a deep, cleansing breath, and just stand in this relaxed position for a moment or two, being aware of how your body feels.

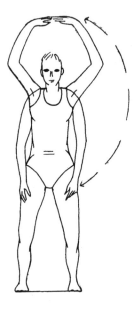

CHI BREATH

Stand with your feet about hip-width apart, facing forwards. 'Soften' your knees and bend them slightly, so that your body and its centre of gravity drop a few inches. Keep your back straight, and do not let your bottom stick out. Let your arms hang easily by your side.

Take a deep, cleansing breath, and relax. With your next in-breath, bring both arms up to the side in a gentle sweep, until they meet above your head with palms facing forward. Let your arms gently fall down the front of your body as you breathe out. Finish the breath by touching the sides of your knees with your hands as you bend forward slightly. Repeat this nice, fluid movement twelve times, with the emphasis on a continuous slow and gentle motion.

Finish by letting your hands gently fall to your sides. Take a deep, cleansing breath, and stand still for a few moments feeling your body and its energy gently settle.

On occasions where mobility becomes more difficult, there are many exercises that you can do while seated. These range from the standard upper-body exercises of lifting and moving the arms, to isotonic exercises where you squeeze and hold the squeeze in the muscles. If you repeat this type of exercise, squeezing, holding and then releasing different muscle groups in turn, you can feel the effects very quickly.

You can also choose to exercise some of your muscles underwater. This is a very good way to work muscles while being safe and supported, and can provide an aerobic work-out if you take part in some type of class or do your exercises in a swimming pool, where you will have the space to incorporate other elements into a gentle routine. Exercising underwater is easier than it is on land, and because there is so much support for the body, you must take care not to overdo it. Take it slowly, like any other exercise, and it will pay dividends.

You can also work muscles in the bath, or in a bowl of water if you need to improve the condition of any area of your body. Simply practise the type of movement that you need to make in the water, and let the warmth and support of the water help you.

Regular exercise of some kind is really important. It improves the circulation, helping you to keep warm, and can be a very enjoyable part of your day. Reward yourself, and improve the condition of your body still further, by using massage to reinforce the work of the exercises. You can massage any part of your body that you can reach. Sometimes what feels good will be simply stroking some part of yourself lightly and lovingly. Other times you might like to use some massage oil, and add a few drops of essential oil to enhance the work still further. Sandalwood essential oil has a particular affinity with older skin, and Frankincense, Rose and Ylang-ylang are also good choices. Jasmine is my all-time favourite, but you can use any oil that you like the smell of and feel good about.

Use to stroke and simply follow the contours of whatever body part you are working on. Make your strokes move down the body, so if you are massaging your arm, direct your strokes from your shoulder down towards your elbow, and then down to your wrist, and over your hands and off the ends of your fingers. Similarly, if working on your legs work down towards your feet and toes.

You can make this a regular treat for yourself – and may also like to consider getting someone else to massage you – a partner, friend, or professional massage therapist.

Breast screening

This is a medical method of checking for any abnormality in the breast tissue and on the chest wall. It is the only medical early detection method for breast cancer. It can be undertaken in the X-ray department of a hospital, or in a special unit. X-rays are taken of each breast by compressing it between two plates. The procedure itself can be uncomfortable but is over quite quickly, taking only a few minutes each time.

The images will be studied by a radiologist, and results normally arrive within a few weeks.

Over 95 per cent of women routinely tested will be given

the all-clear. If a suspect area is found, the next step is a repeat X-ray, often accompanied by an ultrasound examination to give further information. About 1 per cent who have X-rays will go on to have a biopsy. This is where a small sample of tissue is removed and tested for malignancy.

False positive results do occur, and they can be enormously stressful. It is worth considering whether, and how often, to have an X-ray rather than just going along with your GP's directive.

In the UK, all women aged between fifty and sixty-four can be routinely screened every three years. Outside of this age group, screening is undertaken privately or on referral from a GP.

There is no doubt that early detection offers the widest possible choice of treatments. There is an argument that handling the delicate breast tissue in this way and exposing the ageing body to repeated X-rays could be some of the reasons for high detection rates throughout the period of testing. This screening programme costs in excess of £30 million per annum in the UK, a staggering figure compared with the £4 million that the British government spends on research into breast cancer each year.

There are, also, natural alternatives. Skilled practitioners of many branches of healthcare have different ways of assessing the body's energy, and have good diagnostic skills that are less invasive or troublesome to the body.

Family history is important because heredity is a big factor, so too is stress, and a diet that is high in animal fats. There is much that you can do to minimise the impact of these last two in your life: take relatively simple steps like reducing the amount of animal fat you eat, and substitute it with cold-pressed virgin olive oil, and learn some enjoyable ways to relax and manage your stress levels more effectively.

What to Eat Now

It is just as important as ever to ensure optimum nutrition as we grow older. The emphasis of the diet will shift away from larger meals and the need to obtain energy from carbohydrates. It is vital to eat regularly, and to drink sufficient amounts. It may be helpful to place a jug of water, diluted juice or barley water in the fridge or by the sink each day, and then you will be reminded to drink at least that much. Stop drinking at least two hours before bedtime to avoid disturbed sleep.

Now is the time to experiment with new tastes and flavours in order to maintain your interest in food. It is also the occasion to explore the medicinal values of food.

Getting to know the healing effects of what you eat places you in a powerful position to look after your own health and well-being. You can adapt your diet to suit your own changing needs as well as in response to the changing seasons, so that both inner and outer worlds may be in harmony. Eat more foods that are locally grown, and cook in line with the season, eating baked, casseroled and oven-cooked meals during the winter, and fast-grilled and stir-fried food in the warmer months.

Take garlic regularly to enhance your health and in larger amounts to fight any infection. Take fresh garlic in preference to a supplement, and chew fresh parsley or coriander leaves to remove any odour on the breath. This is especially good to take in early autumn, along with a vitamin C supplement, to prepare for the winter.

Mung beans are an easily assimilated source of protein and are also high in fibre. Eat sprouted beans raw or gently stir-fried. Stew the dried beans until soft, then flavour with crushed fresh garlic and ginger, and a little powdered cinnamon and serve with rice for a wonderfully satisfying meal.

Turmeric is useful for eliminating mucus. Add to rice, sprinkle on cooked meals, or use to flavour oil for salad dressing. This is especially useful for fighting colds, and aids sinus conditions and chesty coughs.

Beetroot is a natural liver tonic. Take a little raw, fresh beetroot or a glass of the juice daily to boost digestion and support the liver. It is a useful tonic when feeling sluggish and in need of a boost.

Almonds are a rich source of calcium. These are wonderful for soothing the nervous system and digestion, and will give a sustained and natural energy lift. Take as many as you can hold in your closed fist each morning, soaking for a few minutes before eating to loosen the skin, which can be rubbed off or eaten, according to taste.

Sesame seeds are the tastiest and most versatile source of calcium. Eat them on their own or roasted and mixed with dried fruits. Ground into a paste as tahini, they can be spread in sandwiches and make a wonderful breakfast topping for toast, pancakes or ricecakes. Try also halva, which is sesame seeds ground and mixed into a paste with honey and often flavoured with pistachio nuts.

As we grow older the risk of osteoporosis does not decrease, so maintaining adequate amounts of calcium in the diet is very necessary. We also need to ensure adequate amounts of vitamin C and D.

Take 1g (1,000mg) of vitamin C as a supplement each day to ensure you are having enough. The amount of vitamin C we get from foods varies enormously according to how fresh they are. A 4oz (110g) serving of fresh beansprouts contains more vitamin C than twelve bought oranges. Vitamin D is present in many dairy foods, eggs, fish and fish oils. It is activated by the presence of sunlight on the skin, so time out-doors is essential.

It is worth taking a broad spectrum multivitamin and mineral supplement every winter, in addition to these other ones (see p.23). This will help boost immunity and energy levels during the colder months. Choose a product that is in capsule form for ease of digestion, and favour a time-release formula.

Also consider taking a supplement of ginkgo biloba. This is the nut of one of the oldest trees in existence, and has been highly prized since ancient times. More recently it has been recognised for its effectiveness in improving circulation and enhancing digestion. Its long-term effects include improving the memory, sexual interest, and the assimilation of nutrients.

When appetite is poor, take a tiny piece of peeled fresh ginger root in a cup of hot water half an hour before meals. If this does not stimulate your desire for food, ensure that you take fresh fruit and vegetable juices, and add some powdered slippery elm for adequate nutrition. Make sure that the food is as appealing as it can be – stimulating your sense of beauty by looking lovely, and being nicely presented. Making the effort to lay a tray or to light a candle and put fresh flowers on the table satisfies many senses at once, and can encourage the appetite and make mealtimes a welcome event.

Staying Well

- Soak your feet occasionally and add a few stones to the water. They will top up your mineral levels and playing with them is an excellent exercise to keep your feet supple. Pick them up with your toes and move them across the bowl or transfer them from one foot to another.

Pick up a larger stone between the soles of both feet. Afterwards, let your feet air-dry by supporting your calves on a chair, pouffe or cushions, and gently circling your feet and wriggling your toes until they are quite dry.

If you can reach them comfortably, this is the ideal time to massage your feet with some warmed sesame or olive oil. Add a drop of sandalwood or another essential oil to fragrance the massage and add its own benefits. Afterwards, put on a pair of socks, and let your feet absorb the rest of the oil, helped by the warmth of the socks.

- Make a herbal infusion to cool and refresh the skin. Use this as an all-over rinse after washing, or as a light toner after cleansing the face. Lime flower, lemon balm and fennel are all effective in improving the local circulation and have a gentle but marked toning effect, reducing the appearance of wrinkles and refreshing the skin. Steep one tablespoon (28ml) of the dried herb in ½ pint (290ml) of boiling water, and use within the day to retain the effects of the herbs.
- Osteoporosis, the loss of fleshy protection and weakening muscle strength all make some joints very vulnerable. The highest risk are the wrist, which we use so often, and sometimes overextend when struggling with sticking lids or lifting things, and our hips which bear so much of our weight. Gentle strengthening exercises will help protect most joints, and these can often form part of the overall fitness plan.

Consider a combination of some form of weight training with regular walking for all-round fitness, or learn one of the gentler strengthening exercise forms from the East, like Chi Kung, Chi Dynamics, or T'ai Chi. You can adapt body-building techniques to fit your own needs by using very light substitutes like cans of soup or packets of rice in place of the weights. Use these to ensure that all your muscles get some regular, strengthening exercise.

TO STRENGTHEN THE WRIST

Hold your wrist level, and make sure that it does not bend. Take hold of a small ball or other soft object, and gently squeeze it in your fist. Support your forearm by resting it on a chair arm or on your lap, and repeat the squeezing. This will strengthen the muscles in your forearm and reinforce the wrist. Take care not to overdo it – start slowly, and increase the number of squeezes every day until you are doing this for about two or three minutes at a time. It may seem like a small and simple exercise, but take care to keep the wrist level, and not to make too many repetitions.

Mary consulted me with a sprained wrist, and was extremely frustrated and cross with herself. A very active seventy-two-year-old, she had hurt herself while trying to open a jar, and couldn't get over being that silly. She had already seen her GP, who had strapped the wrist and prescribed some pain killers. Mary said she hated taking any tablets, and that she hadn't taken any all of her life, and wasn't going to start now.

I restrapped her wrist and bound some fresh comfrey leaves inside the dressing. This is a wonderful herb, and its country or common name is Boneknit. It was often bound into wound packings in olden days for its antiseptic and bone-knitting qualities. Mary was as interested in the history and why it would work as she was in the cure itself.

As soon as it was ready to leave behind the support of the strapping, Mary began some hydrotherapy measures to increase circulation to the wrist and speed its full recovery. Every time she passed a sink she held her wrist under the cold tap for three minutes. This simple technique increased the blood supply to the area and further reduced any inflammation. She was also taking a balanced calcium and magnesium supplement – an easy-to-absorb form of calcium.

Once she was feeling strong enough she began strengthening exercises for both wrists. While sitting down she began to gently squeeze a soft ball, keeping her wrist level and her arm well supported. She did this for five minutes, three times a day, and was soon noticing improved strength and confidence in her renewed ability.

TO STRENGTHEN THE HIP

These two exercises can follow each other, or be done at different times each day. Start by standing with your feet a little way apart – about shoulder width – and slowly and rhythmically sway from side to side, lifting your foot up and slightly out to the side as you sway away from it and bear your weight on your outer leg. Then sway back, and lift the other leg as you lean away from it. Keep the swaying gentle, and the movements small, and repeat as often as feels comfortable. It is important not to strain, and this exercise makes a wonderful warm-up for the lower body.

A more specific exercise for the hip area requires you to hold on to either a door handle or a piece of furniture to steady yourself. Stand at right angles to your support, holding on with your right hand, and raise your left foot an inch or two off the floor. Let your right leg support your weight, and steady yourself with the grip of your right hand. Swing your leg very slowly and gently from front to back, using your muscles to control the movement. Keep your knee bent and your foot just a few inches off the ground. Do not let the swing gather any momentum, keep it nice and controlled, lifting your leg behind you by using the muscles around the top of your bottom, and letting your thigh muscles carry your leg forward. This explanation sounds laboured, but the movement itself should be smooth, slow and gentle, and you should be able to feel the muscles all around the hip area working. Aim to achieve about twenty swings and then change to your other leg.

Managing stress

Loneliness, worry, grief and fear of change can all cause their own tremendous stress. Any unexpressed feelings can fester and leave us tense, unhappy, and unwell.

Laughter is a natural de-stressor. A good laugh can relax and massage your entire digestive system, as well as loosening up the shoulders, face and tummy – three classic sites for holding tension. Happiness and laughter have a beneficial effect on all the body's systems, and regular doses are recommended for optimum benefit.

Taking time off from your daily routine to have fun is a legitimate health-enhancing pursuit. Seeing the funny side of things can often be all we need to change a difficult situation into one that we can manage. It will certainly transform physical feelings of discomfort and stiffness into something more free and flexible. It is worth asking yourself when was the last time you had a good, deep, belly-laugh – the side-splitting, uncontrollable, knicker-wetting type. The answer is, probably, too long ago.

Make some time right now to go to see a funny film, or a comedian, to watch a comedy on TV, or get together with friends you know you can have a good time with, read a funny book or cartoon collection, or do whatever makes you laugh.

Alzheimer's disease

This was once known more commonly as early senility or senile dementia. There is a strong link with heavy metals, especially aluminium, so it is important to eliminate these from your kitchen. Switch to a different form of saucepan and limit the times you let tin-foil come in contact with your food. Magnesium and sulphur are both useful in removing aluminium from the system, so increase the amount of these in the diet, and consider taking a magnesium supplement. Good food sources of magnesium include fresh fruit and vegetables, particularly broccoli, and chickpeas. Sulphur-containing foods include eggs, peppers, onions and garlic.

Amalgam dental fillings can leak mercury, and you may consider having them replaced, although the alternatives also have their own hazards. If you have a number of mercury fillings consider following a personalised detox programme, worked out by your practitioner.

Levels of a chemical massage carrier called acetylcholine are found to be quite low when the disease is present. Lecithin can help with this, and again may be taken as a supplement. Good dietary sources include soya beans, wheatgerm, whole grains, fish and brewer's yeast.

It is important to stay on top of things, and treat all symptoms as they occur.

Hair loss

Keep your hair and your scalp healthy from within by ensuring a varied diet that is rich in natural nutrients.

Maintain the blood flow to the scalp by ensuring there are no osteopathic problems in the neck, and that you do not hold too much tension in your shoulders. Massage your head regularly with a mixture of olive and sesame oil and add one drop of essential oil of Rosemary or Thyme. Do this in the morning on a sunny day, and let the sun provide your heat treatment, knowing that the oil will protect the condition of your hair. Otherwise, you can massage the scalp at any time, and wrap in a warm towel to ensure that it is well absorbed. This is also a fantastic conditioner for the hair.

Do not be afraid to press quite firmly on your scalp, using small circular movements with your fingers, and letting the warmth of your hands relax you and encourage the oil's absorption.

Failing eyesight

Exercise your eyes regularly to keep them in the best possible shape. Regularly shift your focus so that your eyes do not tire from spending too long concentrating on any one thing. Do this easily while reading or watching television by looking up and out of the window, then over at the wall, then down to your hands, before returning to your original focus. Repeat this as often as you think of it, but at least once every half-hour.

Exercise the muscles around your eyes on waking each morning by opening your eyes wide for a moment, then make complete circles with your eyes without moving your head. Look down, then to the left as far as you can, up as far as you can, then to the right. On completing the circle, repeat it a few times, then repeat the exercise making anticlockwise circles.

Dental care

Rub your gums regularly with a solution of tincture of Myrrh, sea salt and fresh chopped mint leaves. Make sure your teeth have work to do by keeping raw foods in the diet. When this becomes difficult, take fresh fruit and vegetable juices. Ensure you have regular contact with the earth. Do this by walking barefoot on clean grass or sand, gardening and handling the soil, or simply being out in nature. This strengthens the whole digestive system, including the mouth, and will reinforce the unity of that system.

Hearing

Practise listening to the sounds in silence. We are bombarded by so much noise that hearing needs time to rest and recover each day. If there are problems with the ears, treat with regular applications of garlic oil, and add extra garlic to your diet. To make garlic oil, place five peeled cloves in a small screw-top jar and cover with almond or olive oil. Leave to steep for five days. Prepare this when the moon is waxing or growing for maximum benefit.

Once ready, apply five drops to the outer ear using a small dropper, and plug the ear with cotton wool. Do this before bedtime and leave in overnight, repeating every night for a week. It is easier if you treat one ear at a time. During cold weather, or if chilled, add two cloves to the garlic for steeping.

Sex

You can continue being sexually active for as long as you choose. Advancing years will alter the experience, but then sex is different at every stage of our lives. Lubrication takes longer and tends to be less profuse than it was, although this can simply be an invitation to prolong the foreplay. Pierce a capsule of vitamin E to lubricate the area, or use any other oil, or cocoa butter. The vulva changes with age, along with the rest of the body, and the thinning of the vaginal lips can expose the clitoris a little more than before, making stimulation easier for many women.

Resources

British Society of Research on Ageing School of Biological Sciences, University of Manchester, 3/239 Stopford Building, Oxford Road, Manchester M13 9PT. 0161 275 5252

Carers National Association 20 Glasshouse Yard, London EC1A 4JS. 0171 490 8818

YOUR NATURAL
HEALTHCARE PLAN

Learn your own cycles of health, and allow the seasons to guide you. See if you can connect in some way with the burgeoning, immediateness of spring, and can use that energy to help you clear any blocks to your health or happiness. Learn more about your ability to relax and receive through the long, langourous days of summer. Let the majesty of autumn teach you the richness that is to be found in letting go, and develop trust through the winter months that your strength will sustain you, and that your hopes and dreams are being held, nurtured and transformed ready to bloom in the spring.

Daily cycles

We can reflect the changing cycles of the natural world in our lives by allowing time to adjust to the different patterns of each day.

Begin each morning with a meditation, dedication, or some way of clearing your motivation and setting the tone for the day ahead. This can be as simple as taking a moment to sit still and review your schedule to ensure you have the resources to meet the day's expected demands. Meditation is a wonderful way to re-experience our own inner calm, peace and security, and to make it manifest in our lives. A regular practice is like a gift to the self.

Dedication can take just a moment to stop and voice the thought of devoting your day to your own highest purpose, or committing to follow your heart or your own true self. Or you may prefer to perform a personal ceremony to mark this. Whatever your way of achieving it, this act of clearing your focus and preparing for the day ahead is very effective.

During the day it is most useful to take a complete break from the demands of work or other activities, and concentrate on nourishing yourself. Make your meal-break really time away from whatever you have been doing, and you will return to it renewed and refreshed. The physical appetite and digestive fire both reach their peak at the middle of the day, just like the elemental fire of the sun, so this is a good time for the main meal.

Give yourself time to wind down from work or the 'busy-ness' of the day before becoming involved in the gentler energy of evening. Make some quiet time before bed to allow yourself to relax fully and review your day so that you do not carry any unresolved matters into your dreaming.

Each day is of course a building block towards a whole new approach to your life. And as this develops, you will also want to start looking at some things in the longer term:

DAILY PLAN

- Take some time to yourself on waking, and before bed.
- Eat five portions of fresh fruit and vegetables.
- Take a walk in the fresh air as part of your exercise plan.

WEEKLY PLAN

- Review your health goals and successes.
- Include one new fruit or vegetable in your shopping.

- Give yourself extra support in one area of your life, e.g. a treat if you are feeling low.
- Review the balance of your week – did you make time for yourself and your own pleasure and leisure, make time for others (altruism is a genuine need), and allow yourself time to rest and enjoy life as well as working?

MONTHLY PLAN

- Plan some form of retreat to coincide with your period.
- Perform a breast examination.
- Plan a day-long fast, or fruit diet.
- Adopt a new good health habit, pursuit or activity.

QUARTERLY PLAN

- Review your supplements in line with the seasonal change.
- Plan a body treat – a massage, aromatherapy appointment, or a long walk in the beauty of nature.

YEARLY PLAN

- Plan a full assessment of your health achievements over the last year, and identify your goals for the year ahead.
- Have a holiday.
- Consider a smear test.

FURTHER INFORMATION

To contact the author, for news of trainings and workshops, and for details of her postal Advice Service, please write to:

Belinda Grant Viagas] Belinda is now in Eire
Contact her at
Natural health care
Ballinrobe
Co. Mayo
nhcballinrobe@yahoo.co.uk